THE CLEVELAND CLINIC FOUNDATION
CREATIVE COOKING for RENAL DIETS

First Edition June 1987

Published under exclusive license by
Senay Publishing, Inc.
P.O. Box 397
Chesterland, Ohio 44026

Library of Congress Cataloging-in-Publication Data

The Cleveland Clinic Foundation creative cooking for renal diets.

   Includes index.
   1. Kidneys--Diseases--Diet therapy--Recipes.
2. Large type books. I. Cleveland Clinic Foundation.
Dept. of Nutrition Serives. II. Ellis, Pat
(Pat Weigel) III. Title: Creative cooking for renal
diets.
RC903.C557 1985   641.5'631   87-4575
ISBN 0-941511-00-6 (soft)

THE CLEVELAND CLINIC FOUNDATION
CREATIVE COOKING for RENAL DIETS

by THE CLEVELAND CLINIC FOUNDATION
DEPARTMENT OF NUTRITION SERVICES

Pat Ellis, M.S., R.D.

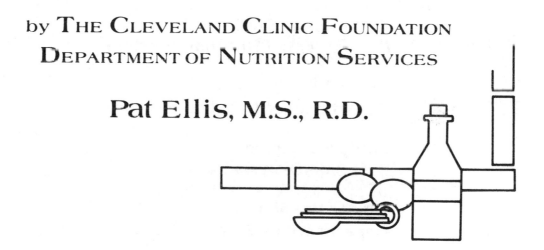

Senay Publishing, Inc.
P.O. Box 397
Chesterland, Ohio 44026

This cookbook has been compiled through the efforts of many individuals at The Cleveland Clinic Foundation. Without the combined contributions and support of these individuals, the publication of this cookbook would not have been possible:

The Cleveland Clinic Foundation
Dialysis Patients

Test Kitchen Staff
Department of Nutrition Services

Clinical Dietitians
Department of Nutrition Services

Kindy Bontempo
East Side Dialysis Center

Ginger Ranallo
Department of Graphic Services

In Appreciation
The Publisher acknowledges his sincere appreciation to Karen Miller Kovach, M.S., R.D. for her assistance in making this edition possible.

NUTRIENT GUIDELINES FOR RENAL EXCHANGES

FOOD GROUP		PROTEIN (G)	SODIUM (MG)	POTASSIUM (MG)	CALORIES
MEAT		8	25	120	75
MILK		4	60	175	80
FRUITS/VEGETABLES		1	5	155	20-40
STARCHES	SALTED	2	150	40	100
	UNSALTED	2	10	40	100
SALTED FATS		0	150	0	100
BEVERAGES		0	0	60	0
CALORIE BOOSTERS		0	0	0	100

The exchanges used follow the Renal Diet Instruction Booklet written by the Northern and Eastern Ohio Council on Renal Nutrition.

Special diets are often difficult to follow because they soon become boring and monotonous. **The Cleveland Clinic Foundation Creative Cooking for Renal Diets** was written to add variety and imagination to your diet. Favorite everyday and special occasion recipes are given with renal exchanges to make your meals more pleasurable and your diet easier to follow.

Some of these recipes may contain formerly forbidden foods, like nuts, chocolate or regular cheese. These foods are calculated into the exchanges listed. Use them only as directed. If you need to gain weight, use those recipes which have salted fats and calorie boosters. Each salted fat or calorie booster listed adds another 100 calories to the serving. If you are trying to lose weight, either avoid those high calorie dishes or cut back on the margarine and oil. Excess fluid weight gains may mean that you are using too much salt. Substitute salt-free margarine or butter in the recipes, try using salt-free breads and starches (rice, noodles and macaroni) and review your diet instruction to see what salty foods you need to avoid.

The Cleveland Clinic Foundation does not endorse any products or brand names. Recipes specifying brand name ingredients are provided for your convenience. Do not substitute ingredients, unless approved by your dietitian.

CONTENTS

BEVERAGES

FLAVORED COFFEES

VIENNA: 1/3 Cup Instant Coffee
2/3 Cup Sugar
2/3 Cup "Coffee Mate"
1/2 Teaspoon Cinnamon

ORANGE: 1/2 Cup Instant Coffee
3/4 Cup Sugar
1 Cup "Coffee Mate"
1/2 Teaspoon Dried Orange Peel

MOCHA: 1/2 Cup Instant Coffee
1/2 Cup Sugar
1 Cup "Coffee Mate"
2 Tablespoons Unsweetened Cocoa

Blend in blender until powdered. For each serving place 2 rounded teaspoons coffee mix in a cup and add boiling water. Makes 20 servings.

Each serving equals: 1 BEVERAGE

COUNT FLUID AS PART OF DAILY FLUID ALLOWANCE

SPICED TEA

1/2 Cup Loose Tea
1-1/2 Tablespoons Dried Orange or Lemon Peel
1 Tablespoon Whole Cloves
1 Teaspoon Cinnamon

Combine tea, dried peel, cloves and cinnamon. Store in an airtight jar. Place 1 teaspoon tea mix in a tea ball and steep in boiling water to taste.

Each serving equals: 1 BEVERAGE

COUNT FLUID AS PART OF DAILY FLUID ALLOWANCE

HOT BUTTERED RUM

1/4 Cup Margarine
1/2 Cup Brown Sugar, Packed*
3 Tablespoons Honey
1-1/2 Teaspoons Rum Extract

3/4 Teaspoon Cinnamon
3/4 Teaspoon Nutmeg
1/8 Teaspoon Cloves

Cream margarine until smooth, gradually beat in brown sugar and continue beating until fluffy. Add honey, rum extract, cinnamon, nutmeg and cloves. Beat until blended. The mix can be stored in a covered container in the refrigerator several weeks or in the freezer for several months. To make one serving, place 1-1/2 tablespoons of the mixture in a cup and stir in 1/2 cup of boiling water, a little at a time until blended. If desired you may add 1 tablespoon rum. Makes 8 servings.

Each serving equals: **1 SALTED FAT**
                               1 BEVERAGE
                               120cc FLUID

* Brown sugar has been specially calculated into this recipe, use it only as directed.

HOT COCOA

1 Teaspoon Unsweetened Cocoa
2 Teaspoons Sugar
3/4 Cup "Coffee Rich"

Mix cocoa powder and sugar in a small saucepan. Add "Coffee Rich", mix well. Heat thoroughly. Serve topped with marshmallows or "Cool Whip", if desired. Makes 1 serving.

Each serving equals: 1 BEVERAGE
3 CALORIE BOOSTERS
180cc FLUID

HOT COCOA MIX

1 Cup "Coffee Mate"
3/4 Cup Sugar
6 Tablespoons Unsweetened Cocoa
1/4 Cup Instant Nonfat Dry Milk

Mix all ingredients, store in tightly covered container. To serve, mix 1 tablespoon hot cocoa mix with boiling water to taste. Makes approximately 38 servings.

1 tablespoon mix equals: 1 BEVERAGE

COUNT FLUID AS PART OF DAILY FLUID ALLOWANCE

HOLIDAY EGGNOG

1-1/2 Cups "Coffee Rich"
2 Eggs
2 Tablespoons Sugar
1-1/2 Teaspoons Vanilla

Combine "Coffee Rich", eggs, sugar and vanilla in blender or beat with electric mixer until well mixed. Chill thoroughly. Serve with a generous sprinkle of nutmeg. Makes six 1/3-cup servings.

Each serving equals: **1 UNSALTED STARCH**
                               80cc FLUID

HOT SPICED WINE

1 Cup Apple Cider
1 Cup Rose' Wine
4 Whole Cloves
1 Stick Cinnamon

Combine ingredients. Simmer to blend flavors. Serve hot. Makes three 2/3-cup servings.

Each serving equals: **1 FRUIT**
                               160cc FLUID

HOT SPICED CRANBERRY PUNCH

1-1/2 Cups Cranberry Juice Cocktail
4 Whole Cloves
2-Inch Stick Cinnamon
1-1/2 Cups Water
3 Tablespoons Sugar
One 6-Ounce Can Frozen Lemonade
3 Thin Orange Slices
6 Maraschino Cherries

Combine cranberry juice, cloves, cinnamon and water in saucepan. Bring to a boil and simmer 5 minutes. Cover, turn off heat and let stand for 5 more minutes. Remove spices. Add sugar and stir until dissolved. Blend in lemonade. Reheat until piping hot. Serve hot, garnished with 1/2 orange slice and cherry on a toothpick. Makes five 3/4-cup servings.

Each serving equals: **1 BEVERAGE**
1 CALORIE BOOSTER
180cc FLUID

COOKIES

ALMOND FLAVORED SHORTBREAD

1 Cup Margarine, Softened
1/2 Cup Sugar
2 Teaspoons Almond Extract
2-1/2 Cup Sifted Flour
Sugar

Beat margarine, sugar and almond extract until light and fluffy. Stir in flour and blend well. Refrigerate, covered, for 2 hours. Divide dough in half. Roll out dough, one half at a time, until 1/2-inch thick. Cut with 2-inch cookie cutter. Place cookies on cookie sheet. Make an indentation in the center of each cookie with the handle of a wooden spoon. Bake at 300° for 25 to 30 minutes. Remove from oven and roll in sugar. Cool. Makes 3-1/2 dozen cookies.

Three cookies equal: **1 SALTED STARCH**
1 CALORIE BOOSTER

BROWNIES

1/2 Cup Sifted Flour	2 Eggs
1/8 Teaspoon Baking Powder	2 Squares Unsweetened
1/2 Cup Margarine, Softened	Chocolate, Melted
1 Cup Sugar	1/2 Teaspoon Vanilla

Mix flour and baking powder; set aside. Cream margarine and sugar until light and fluffy; beat in eggs, 1 at a time, until very light. Beat in melted chocolate and vanilla. Blend in flour mixture just until combined. Pour into lightly greased 8-inch pan, spreading evenly. Bake at 325° for 30 minutes. Cool 10 minutes. With a sharp knife, cut into 12 squares. Cool completely.

Each brownie equals: **1 SALTED STARCH**
                                              1 CALORIE BOOSTER

BROWNIE MIX

4 Cups Sifted Flour
8 Cups Sugar
2-1/2 Cups Unsweetened Cocoa
4 Teaspoons Baking Powder
2 Cups Shortening

Sift together flour, sugar, cocoa and baking powder into a very large bowl. Cut in shortening with pastry blender or two knives. (You can also do it in several batches with a food processor and then remix it all together.) Store in a covered container in a cool place or refrigerator up to 3 months. Makes about 16 cups.

SHORT-CUT BROWNIES

2 Cups Brownie Mix
2 Eggs, Slightly Beaten
1 Teaspoon Vanilla

Combine mix, eggs and vanilla in a bowl, blending well. Mixture will not be smooth. Spread in a greased 8-inch square baking pan. Bake at 350° for 20 to 25 minutes. Cut into 16 squares.

Each brownie equals: 1 SALTED STARCH

CANDY CHIPPERS

1/2 Cup Margarine
1/2 Cup Sugar
1/4 Cup Brown Sugar*
1 Egg
1 Teaspoon Vanilla

1-1/4 Cups Flour
1/2 Teaspoon Baking Soda
1 Cup Chocolate Chips
1/2 Cup Crushed
   Peppermint Candy

Cream margarine, sugars, egg and vanilla until light and fluffy. Combine flour and baking soda; stir into margarine mixture. Fold in chocolate chips and peppermint candy. Drop from teaspoon onto cookie sheets and bake at 375° for 10 minutes. Makes 3 dozen cookies.

Three cookies equal: **1 SALTED STARCH**
                               1 CALORIE BOOSTER

* Brown sugar is high in potassium and is specially calculated into this recipe. Use only as directed.

CHOCOLATE CHIPPERS

Follow recipe for candy chippers omitting crushed peppermint candy. Makes 3 dozen cookies.

Three cookies equal: **1 SALTED STARCH**
                               1 CALORIE BOOSTER

CHRISTMAS SLICES

1 Cup Margarine, at Room Temperature
1/2 Cup Sugar
1 Egg
1/2 Teaspoon Vanilla
2 Cups plus 2 Tablespoons Flour
1/4 Cup (1-1/2 Ounces) Red or Green Tinted Sugar

Beat margarine in a bowl until creamy. Add 1/2 cup sugar, 1/4 cup at a time, beating well after each addition. Add egg and vanilla, beat until light and fluffy. Mix in flour. Cut dough in half. Using lightly floured hands and board; roll each piece into a cylinder about 9 inches long and 1-1/2 inches in diameter. Sprinkle 2 tablespoons of colored sugar on a strip of waxed paper. Using the waxed paper as a sling, gently roll each piece of dough back and forth until it is evenly coated with sugar. (Cylinders now will be approximately 12 inches long, 1 inch in diameter). Wrap dough and chill 6 hours or more. Slice dough as thin as possible then place slices 1 inch apart on ungreased cookie sheets. Bake at 350° for 6 to 8 minutes, until just firm to the touch, but not browned. Remove from oven and transfer to wire racks to cool. Makes about 110 cookies.

Six cookies equal: **1 SALTED STARCH**
                                   1 CALORIE BOOSTER

FROSTED PINEAPPLE COOKIES

6 Tablespoons Margarine
1/2 Cup Sugar
1 Egg
1/2 Cup Undrained Crushed Pineapple
1-1/2 Cups Flour
1/4 Teaspoon Baking Soda
2 Tablespoons Margarine
2 Tablespoons Milk
1 Cup Confectioners' Sugar
1 Teaspoon Vanilla

Beat 6 tablespoons margarine with sugar and egg until fluffy. Stir in pineapple. Mix flour and baking soda; add to margarine mixture. Beat well. Drop by teaspoonsful on cookie sheet. Bake at 350° for 10-12 minutes.

When cool, frost with icing made by mixing 2 tablespoons margarine, milk, confectioners' sugar and vanilla until smooth. Makes 3 dozen.

Three cookies equal: **1 SALTED STARCH**
                               1 CALORIE BOOSTER

GUMDROP JUMBOS

1 Cup Margarine, Softened
1/2 Cup Sugar
1/2 Cup Brown Sugar*
2 Eggs
1 Teaspoon Vanilla

2 Tablespoons Water
2-3/4 Cups Flour
1/2 Teaspoon Soda
3-1/3 Cups Miniature Gumdrops

Cream margarine, sugars, eggs, vanilla and water. Stir in flour and soda. Fold in gumdrops. Drop by tablespoonsful onto cookie sheet. Bake at 375° for 12 to 15 minutes. Makes 3 dozen large cookies.

Two cookies equal: **1 SALTED STARCH**
2 CALORIE BOOSTERS

*Brown sugar is high in potassium and is specially calculated into this recipe. Use only as directed.

JAM BARS

1-1/2 Cups Flour
1/2 Cup Sugar
1/2 Teaspoon Baking Powder
1/2 Cup Margarine
1 Egg

1/4 Cup Milk
1/2 Teaspoon Almond Extract
1 Cup Strawberry or
   Raspberry Jam
1/3 Cup Confectioners' Sugar

Mix flour, sugar and baking powder together, cut margarine into dry ingredients until the mixture has the texture of cornmeal. Add egg, milk and almond extract; mix well. Spread 2/3 of the batter in a 9 x 13-inch pan. Top evenly with jam and drop remaining batter by spoonsful on top. Bake at 400° for 30 minutes. Cool in pan. Cut into 28 bars and sprinkle with confectioners' sugar.

Two bars equal: **1 SALTED STARCH**
                             1 CALORIE BOOSTER

LEMON DROPS

1/2 Cup Margarine
1 Cup Sugar
2 Eggs
1 Teaspoon Vanilla
2 Cups Flour
1/2 Teaspoon Baking Soda
1/4 Cup Lemon Juice

1-1/2 Cups Confectioners' Sugar
2 Teaspoons Water
1/2 Teaspoon Lemon Extract

Cream margarine and sugar until light and fluffy. Add eggs and vanilla and beat well. Mix flour and baking soda; add with lemon juice to margarine mixture. Mix well. Drop by teaspoonsful onto cookie sheet. Bake at 375° for 10-12 minutes.

When cool, frost with icing made by beating confectioners' sugar, water and lemon extract until smooth. Makes 3 dozen.

Two cookies equal: **1 SALTED STARCH**
1 CALORIE BOOSTER

LEMON SQUARES

2 Cups Flour
1/2 Cup Confectioners' Sugar
1 Cup Margarine
4 Eggs
2 Cups Sugar
1/2 Cup Lemon Juice
1/4 Cup Flour
1/2 Teaspoon Baking Powder
2 Tablespoons Confectioners' Sugar

Combine 2 cups flour and 1/2 cup confectioners' sugar. Cut in margarine until mixture is like pie dough. Press into a 9 x 13-inch pan. Bake at 350° for 20 to 25 minutes until light brown. Beat eggs well, add sugar, lemon juice, 1/4 cup flour and baking powder. Mix well. Pour lemon mixture over baked crust and return to oven for 25 minutes. Sprinkle with 2 tablespoons confectioners' sugar, cool and cut into 24 squares.

Each square equals: **1 SALTED STARCH**
                            1 CALORIE BOOSTER

MELTAWAYS

1 Cup Margarine
1/2 Cup Sifted Confectioners'
   Sugar
1-1/2 Cups Flour
1 Teaspoon Vanilla
3/4 Cup Finely Chopped Walnuts*
1 Cup Sifted Confectioners' Sugar

1 Cup Confectioners' Sugar
1/2 Teaspoon Vanilla
1 Teaspoon Milk
Food Coloring

In a large bowl, beat margarine with 1/2 cup confectioners' sugar until light and fluffy. Stir in flour, 1 teaspoon vanilla and nuts, blending well to make a stiff dough. Roll dough, a level teaspoon at a time, into balls between palms of hands. Place 1 inch apart on cookie sheets. Bake at 350° for 15 minutes or until firm. Remove carefully from cookie sheets; while still hot, roll again in 1 cup confectioners' sugar to make a generous white coating.

Make icing by combining 1 cup confectioners' sugar, 1/2 teaspoon vanilla and milk. Divide icing in half, tint each half to desired color. Spread icing on flat side on half the cookies. Press flat sides of uniced cookies to frosted cookies. Makes 3 dozen double cookies.

Two cookies equal: **1 SALTED STARCH**
                            1 CALORIE BOOSTER

* Walnuts are high in potassium. They have been specially calculated into this recipe. Use only as directed.

MOON PIES

1/2 Cup Milk
2 Teaspoons Lemon Juice
1/2 Cup Margarine
1 Cup Sugar
1 Egg
2 Cups Flour
1/3 Cup Unsweetened Cocoa
1 Teaspoon Baking Soda
1/2 Cup Hot Water

2 Tablespoons Margarine
1 Tablespoon Milk
1 Cup Confectioners' Sugar
1 Teaspoon Vanilla or 1/8 Teaspoon Peppermint Extract
Food Coloring

Combine 1/2 cup milk and lemon juice, set aside. Cream 1/2 cup margarine and sugar, add egg and beat well. Add flour and cocoa alternately with baking soda dissolved in hot water and the milk mixture. Drop by large teaspoonsful onto cookie sheet. Bake at 375° for 8 to 10 minutes.

Make icing by combining 2 tablespoons margarine, 1 tablespoon milk, confectioners' sugar and flavoring, beat until creamy. Tint with food coloring if desired. When cookies are cool, fill sandwich style with frosting. Makes 18 sandwich cookies.

Each sandwich cookie equals: **1 SALTED STARCH**
                                      1 CALORIE BOOSTER

RICH ALMOND COOKIES

1 Cup Margarine, Softened
1/2 Cup Sugar
2 Egg Yolks
2 Tablespoons Water
1-1/2 Teaspoons Almond Extract
2-1/2 Cups Sifted Flour

Cream margarine until fluffy. Gradually add sugar and cream together until light and fluffy. Thoroughly mix in egg yolks, water, almond extract and flour. (Dough may be tinted with food color if desired). Force dough through cookie press onto ungreased cookie sheets. Bake at 500° until golden, about 7-10 minutes. Makes 7 dozen cookies.

Five cookies equal: **1 SALTED STARCH**

SCOTTISH SHORTBREAD

1 Cup Margarine, Softened
1/2 Cup Sugar
1/2 Teaspoon Vanilla
2-1/2 Cups Flour

Line the bottoms of two 8-inch round cake pans with waxed paper and set aside. Cream margarine, sugar and vanilla until light and fluffy. Beat in flour, 1/2 cup at a time, until well mixed. Divide dough in half, pat each half evenly into pans. Prick dough all over with a fork to prevent bubbles from forming during baking. Bake for 1 hour at 275° until pale and golden. (Do not brown). Cool in pans for 10 minutes, then remove from pans and cut each into 8 wedges. Makes 16 cookies.

Each cookie equals: **1 SALTED STARCH**
                            1 CALORIE BOOSTER

SNICKERDOODLES

1 Cup Margarine
1-1/2 Cups Sugar
2 Eggs
2-3/4 Cups Flour
2 Teaspoons Cream of Tartar
1 Teaspoon Soda
2 Tablespoons Sugar
2 Teaspoons Cinnamon

Cream margarine and 1-1/2 cups sugar until light and fluffy. Add eggs and beat well. Mix flour, cream of tartar and soda. Add to margarine mixture, mix well. Form into 1-1/4-inch balls. Roll in mixture of 2 tablespoons sugar and 2 teaspoons cinnamon. Place on cookie sheets. Bake at 400° for 8-10 minutes. Makes 5 dozen.

Two cookies equal: **1 SALTED STARCH**

TEA CAKES

1 Cup Margarine, Softened
1/2 Cup Confectioners' Sugar
1 Tablespoon Water
1 Teaspoon Vanilla
2-1/4 Cups Sifted Flour
1 Cup Confectioners' Sugar

Cream margarine and 1/2 cup confectioners' sugar until light and fluffy. Add water and vanilla, mix well. Gradually add flour, beating until well mixed. Chill dough for 30 minutes or until firm. Roll dough into 1-inch balls. Place on cookie sheets. Bake at 400° for 10 minutes or until light brown on bottom. Cool on wire racks for 10 minutes and roll in remaining 1 cup confectioners' sugar. When completely cool, roll again in remaining confectioners' sugar. Makes 4 dozen cookies.

Three cookies equal: **1 SALTED STARCH**
                             1 CALORIE BOOSTER

THUMBPRINT COOKIES

1 Teaspoon Vanilla
1/4 Teaspoon Lemon Extract
1/2 Cup Margarine
1/4 Cup Sugar
1 Egg Yolk
1 Cup Sifted Flour
Raspberry Jam

Cream vanilla and lemon extract into margarine. Add sugar gradually; beat in egg yolk. Stir in flour. Shape into small balls. Place on cookie sheet and make a dent in each cookie with floured thumb. Fill "dents" with 1/2 teaspoon jam. Bake at 400° for 15 minutes. Makes 24 cookies.

Three cookies equal: **1 SALTED STARCH**
                              1 CALORIE BOOSTER

SNACKS AND SWEETS

HONEY ORANGE SNACK BARS

1/4 Cup Margarine
1/4 Cup Honey
2 Tablespoons Sugar

2-3 Teaspoons Grated
Orange Peel
3 Cups Puffed Rice

Combine margarine, honey, sugar and orange peel in a 1-quart saucepan. Bring to a boil over medium-high heat, stirring occasionally. Simmer over medium heat for 2 minutes, stirring constantly. Pour honey mixture over puffed rice. Mix well. Press firmly into a greased 8-inch square baking pan. Cut into 30 bars. Chill several hours until firm. Store in tightly covered container in refrigerator. Makes 30 bars.

Three bars equal: **1 CALORIE BOOSTER**

OLD-FASHIONED POPCORN BALLS

2 Cups Sugar
1-1/2 Cups Water
1/2 Cup Light Corn Syrup

1 Teaspoon Vinegar
1 Teaspoon Vanilla
5 Quarts Unsalted Popped Popcorn

Grease the sides of a saucepan. Combine sugar, water, cornstarch and vinegar in saucepan. Cook to hard ball stage (250°). Stir in vanilla. Pour slowly over popped corn, stirring just to mix well. Butter hands lightly, shape mixture into balls. Makes 20 balls.

Each popcorn ball equals: **1 CALORIE BOOSTER**

RICE KRISPIE MARSHMALLOW SQUARES

2 Tablespoons Margarine
2 Cups Miniature Marshmallows
2 Cups "Rice Krispies"

Melt margarine in saucepan. Add marshmallows and stir until almost melted. Pour over "Rice Krispies"; mix well. Press into lightly greased 9-inch square pan. Cool and cut into 16 squares.

Five squares equal: 1 SALTED STARCH
                             1 SALTED FAT

PUFFED RICE BRITTLE

1-1/2 Cups Sugar
3 Cups Puffed Rice

Carefully melt sugar in heavy skillet over medium high heat. Stir constantly to prevent scorching. When sugar is melted and carmel colored, mix in puffed rice. Stir quickly to coat puffed rice. Pour into lightly greased 8 x 12-inch pan. Cool. Cut or break into about 30 pieces.

Two pieces equal: 1 CALORIE BOOSTER
       or
10 pieces equal: 1 UNSALTED STARCH
                            8 CALORIE BOOSTERS

BLONDE FUDGE

2 Cups Sugar
1/2 Cup Milk
1/2 Cup Light Cream
1 Tablespoon Light Corn Syrup
1 Tablespoon Margarine
1 Teaspoon Vanilla
1/4 Cup Chopped Candied Cherries

Grease the sides of a 2-quart saucepan. In it combine sugar, milk, cream and corn syrup. Cook over medium heat, stirring constantly, until sugar dissolves and mixture boils. Cook to soft ball stage (238°). Immediately remove from heat; cool to luke warm (110°) without stirring. Add margarine and vanilla. Beat vigorously until fudge stiffens and loses its gloss. Quickly stir in candied cherries. Spread in greased 9 x 5-inch pan. Score while warm; cut into 24 pieces when firm.

Each piece equals: 1 CALORIE BOOSTER

(LIMIT TO 4 PIECES A DAY)

BUTTERSCOTCH WAFERS

1/2 Cup Sugar
1/4 Cup White Corn Syrup
1/4 Cup Water
1 Tablespoon Margarine
1/2 Teaspoon Vanilla Extract

In a 2-quart saucepan, combine sugar, corn syrup and water. Cook over low heat, stirring, until sugar is dissolved. Continue gentle cooking, without stirring to 265° (very hard ball stage). Add margarine and cook to 290° (brittle stage). Remove from heat, add vanilla. Drop from teaspoon onto greased pan. When firm remove with spatula. Makes 2 dozen.

Three pieces equal: **1 CALORIE BOOSTER**

CHOCOLATE FUDGE

2/3 Cup "Coffee Rich"
1-2/3 Cups Sugar
2 Cups Miniature Marshmallows
1-1/2 Cups "Baker's Imitation Chocolate Chips"
1 Teaspoon Vanilla

Combine "Coffee Rich" and sugar in a large, heavy saucepan. Bring to a rolling boil, reduce heat to medium. Stir constantly and continue a rolling boil for 5 minutes. Remove from heat and add marshmallows, chocolate chips, and vanilla. Beat with electric mixer until smooth. Pour into a buttered 9-inch pan. Cool and cut into 36 squares.

Two pieces equal: **1 CALORIE BOOSTER**
               (LIMIT TO 4 PIECES A DAY)
       or
8 pieces equal: **1 UNSALTED STARCH**
               5 CALORIE BOOSTERS

CREAM CHEESE CANDY

3 Ounces Cream Cheese
2-3/4 Cups Sifted Confectioners' Sugar
1/4 to 1/2 Teaspoon Black Walnut Extract or Other Flavoring

Beat cream cheese with electric mixer or by hand until smooth. Add confectioners' sugar, a little at a time and beat well. Add flavoring and mix well. Drop by spoonsful onto squares of plastic wrap and wrap individually. Makes 21 pieces.

Three pieces equal: **1/2 SALTED STARCH**
                                    2 CALORIE BOOSTERS

HARD CANDY

Confectioners' Sugar
3-3/4 Cups Sugar
1-1/2 Cups Light Corn Syrup
1 Cup Water
1 Teaspoon Flavoring Oil*
Desired Food Coloring*

Sprinkle 18 x 24-inch strip of heavy duty aluminum foil with powdered sugar. Mix sugar, corn syrup and water in a large, heavy saucepan. Stir over medium heat until sugar dissolves. Boil, without stirring, until temperature reaches 310° or until drops of syrup form hard and brittle threads in cold water. Remove from heat. Stir in flavoring oil and coloring. Pour onto foil. Cool; break into pieces. Store in airtight container. Makes 2-1/4 pounds (36 ounces).

One ounce equals: **1 CALORIE BOOSTER**

*Suggested flavor and color combinations:

PEPPERMINT	PINK
CINNAMON	RED
LEMON	YELLOW
WINTERGREEN	LIGHT GREEN
CHERRY	RED
BUTTERSCOTCH	YELLOW

HONEY TAFFY

1 Cup Sugar
3 Tablespoons Cornstarch
1/2 Cup Water
2/3 Cup Honey

Combine sugar, cornstarch, water and honey in a 2-quart saucepan. Cook slowly, stirring constantly, until sugar dissolves. Cook to hard ball stage (265°) without stirring. Remove from heat, pour into lightly greased shallow pan. Cool until comfortable to handle. Grease hands; gather taffy into a ball and pull. When candy is light in color and gets hard to pull, cut in half. Pull each piece into a long strand about 1/2-inch thick. With buttered scissors, quickly snip into bite-size pieces. Wrap each piece in waxed paper. Makes 40 pieces.

Three pieces equal: 1 CALORIE BOOSTER

PEANUT BUTTER FUDGE

2 Cups Sugar
3/4 Cup Milk
2 Tablespoons Margarine
1 Teaspoon Vanilla
1/4 Cup Low-Sodium Peanut Butter

Heat sugar, milk and margarine in saucepan; cook slowly, stirring until the sugar is dissolved. Continue cooking, stirring until soft ball stage is reached (238°).

Remove from heat and set aside to cool without stirring. When candy has cooled to lukewarm, add vanilla and peanut butter. Beat fudge until thick and creamy and it loses its sticky consistency. Pour into greased pan. Cool and cut into 20 pieces.

Two pieces equal: **1 UNSALTED STARCH**
                             1 CALORIE BOOSTER

PENUCHE

2 Tablespoons Margarine
2 Cups Sugar
1/2 Cup Milk

1/2 Cup Light Corn Syrup
1 Teaspoon Vanilla

Grease sides of heavy 2-quart saucepan with margarine. Combine remaining margarine, sugar, milk and corn syrup. Heat over medium heat, stirring constantly, until sugars dissolve and mixture comes to a boil. Cook to soft ball stage (238°), stirring only if necessary. Immediately remove from heat and cool to lukewarm (110°) **DO NOT STIR.** Add vanilla. Beat vigorously until candy becomes very thick and starts to lose its gloss. Pour into a lightly greased pan. Cut into 36 squares when warm.

Two pieces equal: **1 CALORIE BOOSTER**

PENUCHE VARIATIONS

COFFEE PENUCHE	-And 1 heaping teaspoon instant coffee with milk.
ORANGE PENUCHE	Cut 1/3 cup candied orange peel into fine bits and add with vanilla.
GINGER PENUCHE	-Cut 1-1/2 tablespoons candied ginger into fine bits and add with vanilla.
CHERRY PENUCHE	-Cut 1/3 cup candied cherries into fine bits and add with vanilla.
MAPLE OR WALNUT FLAVORED PENUCHE	-Substitute 1/2 teaspoon maple or black walnut for vanilla.

Two pieces equal: **1 CALORIE BOOSTER**

WALNUT PENUCHE-   Add 1/2 cup chopped walnuts* with vanilla.

Five pieces equal: **1 UNSALTED STARCH**
3 CALORIE BOOSTERS

* Walnuts are high in potassium and contribute to the protein in this recipe. Instead of counting as a calorie booster, a serving of unsalted starch must be counted to cover the increased protein and potassium.

QUICK BREADS

QUICK BREADS

HAWAIIAN QUICK BREAD

1/3 Cup Sugar
1/3 Cup Margarine
2 Eggs
2 Cups Flour

3 Teaspoons Baking Powder
1 Cup Crushed Pineapple,
Undrained

Beat sugar and margarine until light and fluffy. Add eggs and mix well. Mix flour and baking powder together. Combine sugar and flour mixtures. Blend. Add pineapple, mix to combine. Pour into greased 9 x 5-inch pan. Bake at 350° for 1 hour. Cut into 20 slices.

Each slice equals: **1 SALTED STARCH**

HOLIDAY CRANBERRY BREAD

2 Cups Flour
1 Cup Sugar
1 Tablespoon Orange Peel
1-1/2 Teaspoons Baking Powder
1/2 Teaspoon Baking Soda

3/4 Cup Orange Juice
2 Tablespoons Melted Margarine
1 Egg
1 Cup Chopped Cranberries
1/2 Cup Chopped Nuts*

Combine flour, sugar, orange peel, baking powder and baking soda. Add orange juice, margarine and egg. Mix quickly. Stir in cranberries and nuts. Pour into greased 9 x 5-inch loaf pan. Bake at 325° for 45 to 55 minutes. Slice into 20 slices.

Each slice equals: **1 SALTED STARCH**

* Nuts are high in potassium. They have been specially calculated into this recipe. Use only as directed.

LEMON TEA BREAD

2 Cups Flour
1-1/2 Teaspoons Baking Powder
1/2 Cup Margarine
1 Cup Sugar
2 Eggs

1/3 Cup Milk
1/2 Cup Walnuts*
2 Teaspoons Lemon Peel
1/4 Cup Lemon Juice
1/3 Cup Sugar

Mix flour and baking powder; set aside. Beat margarine and sugar until light and fluffy. Add eggs one at a time, beating well after each addition; beat until light and fluffy. Mix in flour and milk alternately; beat just until combined. Stir in nuts and lemon peel. Spoon into greased 9 x 5-inch loaf pan. Bake at 350° for 55 to 60 minutes or until done.

Combine lemon juice and sugar in a small pan, cook, stirring 1 minute, or until syrupy. Pour evenly over bread as soon as it is removed from oven. Let cool in pan 10 minutes. Remove from pan; let cool completely on a wire rack. Cut into 20 slices.

Each slice equals: **1 SALTED STARCH**
                            1 CALORIE BOOSTER

* Walnuts are high in potassium. They have been specially calculated into this recipe. Use only as directed.

PUMPKIN BREAD

2 Cups Flour
2 Teaspoons Baking Powder
1/2 Teaspoon Baking Soda
1 Teaspoon Cinnamon
1/2 Teaspoon Nutmeg

1 Cup Pumpkin
1 Cup Sugar
1/2 Cup Milk
2 Eggs
1/4 Cup Margarine, Softened

Combine flour, baking powder, baking soda, cinnamon and nutmeg. Mix pumpkin, sugar, milk and eggs together in mixing bowl. Add dry ingredients and softened margarine, mix until well blended. Spread in well greased 9 x 5-inch loaf pan. Bake at 350° for 55 minutes or until done. Cut into 20 slices.

Each slice equals: **1 SALTED STARCH**

STRAWBERRY BREAD

1-1/2 Cups Flour
1/2 Teaspoon Baking Soda
1-1/2 Teaspoons Cinnamon
1 Cup Sugar
1 Egg, Beaten

1/2 Cup Plus 2 Tablespoons Oil
One 10-Ounce Package Frozen,
   Sliced Strawberries, Thawed
Red Food Coloring (Optional)

Combine flour, baking soda, cinnamon and sugar. Add egg and oil, stirring only until dry ingredients are moistened. Stir in strawberries. Blend in a few drops of red food coloring, if desired. Spoon batter into a lightly greased 8 x 4-inch loaf pan. Bake at 350° for 1 hour. Let stand overnight before slicing. Slice into 15 slices.

Each slice equals: **1 UNSALTED STARCH**
                           1 CALORIE BOOSTER

QUICK CINNAMON BREAD

1/2 Cup Sugar
1 Egg
1-1/4 Cups "Coffee Rich"
3 Cups Biscuit Mix
  (See Recipe Page D 12)

2 Tablespoons Cinnamon
1/2 Cup Sugar
1/2 Cup Confectioners' Sugar
1 Tablespoon Milk

Mix 1/2 cup sugar, egg, "Coffee Rich" and biscuit mix. Beat vigorously 30 seconds. (Batter will be lumpy.) Pour 1/3 of batter into greased 9 x 5-inch loaf pan, sprinkle generously with cinnamon mixed with 1/2 cup sugar. Add 1/3 more batter and cinnamon sugar mixture, repeat with remaining batter and cinnamon sugar. Cut with knife swirling through batter. Bake at 350° for 45 to 50 minutes until done. Cool slightly. Make glaze by mixing 1/2 cup confectioners' sugar and 1 tablespoon milk. Spread on loaf. Slice into 20 slices.

Each slice equals: 1 SALTED STARCH

ZUCCHINI BREAD

1-1/2 Cups Flour
1 Teaspoon Cinnamon
1/2 Teaspoon Baking Soda
1/2 Teaspoon Baking Powder
1 Cup Sugar
1/2 Cup Oil

2 Eggs
2 Teaspoons Lemon Peel
1 Cup Grated, Unpeeled Zucchini
1/4 Cup Raisins
1/2 Cup Chopped Walnuts*

Mix flour, cinnamon, baking soda and baking powder together. Combine sugar, oil and eggs in large mixing bowl, mix until smooth. Combine lemon peel, zucchini, raisins and walnuts in separate mixing bowl. Add dry ingredients to sugar mixture. Mix until smooth. Add zucchini mixture and stir until well mixed. Pour into greased and floured 9 x 5-inch pan. Bake at 350° 60 minutes or until done. Cool 10 minutes, remove from pan and continue cooling on wire rack. Cut into 20 slices.

Each slice equals: **1 SALTED STARCH**

*Walnuts are high in potassium. They have been specially calculated into this recipe. Use them only as directed.

HOT MUFFINS

1-1/2 Cups Flour
2 Teaspoons Baking Powder
1/2 Cup Sugar

1 Egg
1 Cup Milk
1/4 Cup Oil

Mix flour, baking powder and sugar. Beat egg until frothy, stir in milk and oil. Pour milk mixture into flour mixture, stir quickly just until mixed (batter will still be lumpy). Fill 16 muffin cups equally. Bake at 425° for 25 minutes or until done. Serve hot. Makes 16 muffins.

Each muffin equals: **1 UNSALTED STARCH**

APPLE MUFFINS

Make hot muffins, add 1/2 teaspoon cinnamon with flour and 1 cup grated raw (unpared) apple with shortening. Sprinkle muffins with mixture of 2 tablespoons sugar and 1/2 teaspoon cinnamon and bake. Makes 16 muffins.

Each muffin equals: **1 UNSALTED STARCH**

JELLY-FILLED MUFFINS

Make hot muffins, fill muffin cups half full. Top with a teaspoon of jelly or marmalade. Top with remaining batter and bake. Makes 16 muffins.

Each muffin equals: **1 UNSALTED STARCH**

BLUEBERRY CAKE MUFFINS

2 Cups Flour
1-1/2 Teaspoons Baking Powder
1/2 Cup Margarine, Softened
1 Cup Sugar
2 Eggs

1 Teaspoon Vanilla
1/2 Cup Milk
1 Cup Blueberries
2 Tablespoons Confectioners'
  Sugar

Preheat oven to 375°. Line 18 muffin cups with paper liners. Mix flour with baking powder and set aside. In a large bowl beat margarine, sugar, eggs and vanilla until light and fluffy. Add milk and flour mixture. Beat just until smooth. Gently fold in blueberries (drain well if canned). Divide muffin batter evenly into muffin cups. Bake 20 to 25 minutes, until golden brown. Cool slightly. Serve warm or cold, sprinkled with confectioners' sugar. Makes 18 muffins.

Each muffin equals: **1 SALTED STARCH**

CORN MUFFINS

1 Cup Flour   1 Egg, Beaten
2 Tablespoons Sugar   1/4 Cup Oil
3 Teaspoons Baking Powder   1 Cup Milk
1 Cup Yellow Cornmeal

Line 18 muffin cups with paper liners. Mix flour, sugar, baking powder and cornmeal in large bowl. In medium bowl, mix egg, oil and milk. Pour milk mixture into flour mixture all at once; stir quickly with fork until all ingredients are just moistened (batter will be lumpy). Quickly dip batter into muffin pans. Bake at 425° for 15 minutes or until golden. Serve hot.

Each muffin equals: 1 SALTED STARCH

STREUSEL-TOPPED MUFFINS

TOPPING:
- 1/4 Cup Brown Sugar*
- 1/4 Cup Flour
- 2 Tablespoons Margarine
- 2 Teaspoons Cinnamon

BATTER:
- 1-1/3 Cup Flour
- 1-1/2 Teaspoons Baking Powder
- 1/4 Cup Margarine
- 1/2 Cup Sugar
- 1 Egg
- 1/2 Cup Milk

Preheat oven to 375°. Line 14 muffin cups with paper liners.

Make Topping: Mix brown sugar, flour, margarine, and cinnamon until crumbly.

Make Batter: Mix flour and baking powder, set aside. Beat margarine until fluffy, beat in sugar, then egg until light and fluffy. Blend in milk, then flour, just until combined. Divide evenly into 14 muffin cups. Sprinkle topping over each muffin. Bake 15 to 18 minutes. Cool slightly, serve warm. Makes 14 muffins.

Each muffin equals: 1 SALTED STARCH

* Brown sugar has been specially calculated into this recipe. Use only as directed.

BAKING POWDER BISCUITS

2 Cups Flour
3 Teaspoons Baking Powder
1/3 Cup Shortening
3/4 Cup Milk

Mix flour and baking powder, cut in shortening until mixture resembles coarse oatmeal. Pour in milk and stir quickly with a fork. Turn dough out on lightly floured board, knead 10 times. Gently roll out dough and cut into 12 biscuits. Bake at 450° for 10 to 12 minutes or until golden brown.

Each biscuit equals: 1 SALTED STARCH

CINNAMON PINWHEELS

1 Recipe Baking Powder Biscuits
(See recipe page D 10)
1/4 Cup Margarine, Melted
1 Teaspoon Cinnamon
3 Tablespoons Sugar

1 Tablespoon Margarine
1 Cup Confectioners' Sugar
1/2 Teaspoon Vanilla
1-2 Tablespoons Milk

Roll out dough to 8 x 10-inch rectangle. Brush with melted margarine. Mix cinnamon and sugar, sprinkle evenly over dough. Roll up jelly-roll fashion, starting with 10-inch side. Cut into 12 slices and bake, cut side down, on a cookie sheet at 450° for 10 to 12 minutes. Make icing by combining margarine, confectioners' sugar and vanilla with enough milk to make a stiff icing. (Icing will melt when put on hot biscuits.) Ice while biscuits are hot and serve immediately.

Each biscuit equals: **1 SALTED STARCH**
                              1 CALORIE BOOSTER

BISCUIT MIX

3 Cups Flour
2 Tablespoons Baking Powder
1/3 Cup Shortening

Mix ingredients until thoroughly combined. Store tightly in refrigerator. Makes 3-3/4 cups. Keeps at least 4 weeks in the refrigerator.

QUICK BISCUITS

1/4 to 1/3 Cup Milk
1 Cup Biscuit Mix

Add milk to biscuit mix and stir with a fork. Dough should be soft and slightly sticky. Knead on floured surface about 10 times. Roll out and cut into 6 biscuits. Bake 10 to 12 minutes at 450° until golden brown.

Each biscuit equals: 1 SALTED STARCH

APPLE CHEESE-FILLED ROLLS

2 Cups Biscuit Mix (See Recipe Page D 12)
1 Cup Sour Cream
One 8-Ounce Package Cream Cheese, Softened
1/3 Cup Sugar
1 Tablespoon Grated Orange Rind
1-1/2 Cups Thinly Sliced, Pared Apples
1/4 Cup Confectioners' Sugar
1-2 Teaspoons Orange Juice

Mix biscuit mix and sour cream until soft dough forms. Turn dough out onto floured board and kneed until smooth, about 20 times. Divide in half. Roll each half into a 9-inch square. Cut into nine 3-inch squares. Place on cookie sheets. Mix cream cheese, sugar and orange peel. Place 2 apple slices on center of each square; top with 1 tablespoon cream cheese mixture. Bring 2 opposite corners of dough to center of each square, overlapping tightly, pinch well. Bake at 400°, until crust is golden brown, approximately 12 to 15 minutes. Cool slightly and drizzle with mixture of confectioners' sugar and orange juice. Makes 18 rolls.

Each roll equals: 1 SALTED STARCH

ONION PARSLEY BUTTERFINGERS

2 Cups Biscuit Mix (See Recipe Page D 12)
1 Egg
1/2 Cup Milk
1/2 Cup Margarine
2 Tablespoons Onion Flakes
1 Tablespoon Parsley

Combine biscuit mix, egg and milk; beat vigorously 20 strokes. Turn dough out on lightly floured surface and knead lightly 1/2 minute; roll out in 12 x 8-inch rectangle and cut with floured knife in 3 x 1-inch fingers. Melt margarine in jelly-roll pan in 450° oven. Lay fingers in margarine; turn once to coat both sides and arrange side by side in pan. Sprinkle with mixture of onion and parsley flakes and bake about 8 minutes or until golden brown. Remove to rack. Serve warm. Makes 32.

Two butterfingers equal: 1 SALTED STARCH

APPLESAUCE RAISIN COFFEE CAKE

2 Cups Biscuit Mix
  (See Recipe Page D 12)
1 Cup Applesauce
1/2 Cup Sugar
1/4 Cup Brown Sugar*
1/4 Cup Oil
1/2 Teaspoon Cinnamon
1/2 Teaspoon Nutmeg
1/8 Teaspoon Cloves

2 Eggs
1/2 Cup Raisins

TOPPING:
1/4 Cup Sugar
2 Tablespoons Biscuit Mix
2 Tablespoons Margarine
2 Teaspoons Cinnamon

Mix biscuit mix, applesauce, sugars, oil, spices and eggs in 9 x 9-inch pan. Stir in raisins. Combine topping ingredients until crumbly. Sprinkle over coffee cake. Bake at 350° for 35 to 40 minutes. Makes 12 servings.

Each serving equals: **1 SALTED STARCH**
                             1/2 FRUIT
                             1 CALORIE BOOSTER

* Brown sugar is high in potassium. It has been specially calculated into this recipe. Use only as directed.

BLUEBERRY KUCHEN

2 Tablespoons Margarine   1 Teaspoon Vanilla
1/2 Cup Sugar   1 Cup Blueberries
1 Egg   3/4 Cup Flour
1/2 Cup Milk   1/2 Cup Sugar
1 Cup Flour   1/4 Cup Margarine
2 Teaspoons Baking Powder

Cream 2 tablespoons margarine and 1/2 cup sugar; add egg, beat well. Add milk, 1 cup flour, baking powder and vanilla and mix well. Pour batter into greased 8 x 8-inch pan. Sprinkle blueberries (drain well, if canned) over batter. Combine 3/4 cup flour, 1/2 cup sugar and 1/4 cup margarine until crumbly. Sprinkle over blueberries. Bake at 375° for 25 to 30 minutes. Cut into 16 pieces.

Each piece equals: **1 SALTED STARCH**

CRANBERRY KUCHEN

Substitute 1 cup fresh or frozen cranberries coarsely chopped and mixed with 1/4 cup sugar for blueberries.

GERMAN COFFEE CAKE

BATTER:
- 1 Cup Flour
- 1/3 Cup Sugar
- 1/8 Teaspoon Nutmeg
- 2 Teaspoons Baking Powder
- 1/2 Cup Milk
- 1 Egg
- 2 Tablespoons Margarine, Melted

TOPPING:
- 1/3 Cup Sugar
- 3 Tablespoons Flour
- 1/2 Teaspoon Cinnamon
- 1/3 Cup Brown Sugar*
- 3 Tablespoons Margarine, Melted

Mix 1 cup flour, 1/3 cup sugar, nutmeg and baking powder. Add milk, egg and 2 tablespoons margarine. Mix well. Pour into 9 x 9-inch greased baking dish. Mix 1/3 cup sugar, 3 tablespoons flour, cinnamon, brown sugar and 3 tablespoons margarine. Spoon over batter, making indentations into batter so some of the topping sinks down into coffee cake. Bake at 350° for 20 to 25 minutes. Serve warm. Makes 12 servings.

Each serving equals: **1 SALTED STARCH**
1 CALORIE BOOSTER

* Brown sugar is high in potassium. It has been specially calculated into this recipe. Use only as directed.

APPLE OVEN PANCAKE

1 Tablespoon Margarine
2 Tablespoons Sugar
1/4 Teaspoon Cinnamon
1 Cup Peeled, Cored, Diced Apples
1/4 Teaspoon Grated Lemon Rind
2 Egg Whites
2 Tablespoons Sugar
2 Egg Yolks
3 Tablespoons Milk
3 Tablespoons Flour
1/4 Teaspoon Baking Powder
1 Tablespoon Sugar

Melt margarine in 9-inch pie plate or ovenproof skillet. Mix 2 tablespoons sugar with cinnamon, apple and lemon rind; set aside. Beat egg whites until frothy, gradually add 2 tablespoons sugar and continue beating until stiff; set aside. Beat egg yolks until light, add milk, flour and baking powder, beat until smooth. Fold in apples and beaten egg whites. Spread batter in pie plate. Sprinkle with 1 tablespoon sugar. Bake at 400° 12 to 15 minutes, until set. Cool 3 to 4 minutes. Serve immediately, plain or with jam, honey or imitation maple syrup. Makes 2 servings.

Each serving equals: **1 OUNCE MEAT**
1 SALTED STARCH
1 SALTED FAT
1 CALORIE BOOSTER

POPOVER PANCAKE

1/4 Cup Margarine
1/2 Cup Flour
1/2 Cup Milk
2 Eggs
Dash Cinnamon or Nutmeg
3 Tablespoons Confectioners' Sugar

Melt margarine in pie pan. Beat flour, milk, eggs and cinnamon or nutmeg until smooth. Pour into pie pan containing margarine. Bake at 375° for 15 minutes until lightly browned. Remove from oven and sprinkle with confectioners' sugar. Return to oven and bake for a few minutes more. Serve immediately with thawed frozen, sweetened strawberries or other sweetened fruit from FRUIT LIST. Makes 2 servings.

Each serving equals: **1 OUNCE MEAT**
                              1 UNSALTED STARCH
                              1/2 MILK
                              2 SALTED FATS

1/2 cup frozen sweetened
strawberries equals: **1 FRUIT**

HUNGARIAN PANCAKES

1 Egg
3/4 Cup Flour
2 Cups "Coffee Rich"
1 Teaspoon Sugar
1 Teaspoon Margarine

Mix egg, flour, "Coffee Rich" and sugar together well with rotary beater. Let batter stand 30 minutes. Melt 1 teaspoon margarine in 9-inch skillet, coat the bottom of the pan lightly. Pour 1/4 cup batter into hot skillet. Quickly tip skillet so batter covers the bottom of the whole pan. Cook over low heat until browned on one side. Transfer to warm plate. Spread with jam, honey or imitation maple syrup. Roll up. Sprinkle with powdered sugar. Repeat with remaining batter, adding more margarine as needed. Serve at once. Makes 10 pancakes.

One pancake equals: **1 UNSALTED STARCH**
            or
Five pancakes equal: **1/2 OUNCE MEAT**
                                  2 UNSALTED STARCHES
                                  2 CALORIE BOOSTERS

PANCAKES

1 Cup Flour	1 Egg, Beaten
2 Teaspoons Baking Powder	1 Cup Milk
2 Tablespoons Sugar	3 Tablespoons Margarine, Melted

Mix flour, baking powder and sugar. Mix beaten egg, milk and melted margarine. Pour into flour mixture all at once. Mix until just combined (batter will be lumpy). Heat skillet or griddle to 425°. Use a scant 1/4 cup batter for each pancake. Makes ten 4-inch pancakes. Serve with margarine and imitation maple syrup.

One pancake equals: 1 SALTED STARCH
       or
Five pancakes equal: 1/2 OUNCE MEAT
                     1 MILK
                     2 SALTED STARCHES
                     1 SALTED FAT

BLUEBERRY PANCAKES

Add 1 cup blueberries (drain, if canned) to pancake batter, fold in carefully, being careful not to break the berries. Cook and serve as directed above.

FRENCH TOAST

2 Eggs
3/4 Cup Milk
6 Slices Bread

Mix egg and milk together and pour into a shallow bowl. Dip slices of bread into mixture, turn to coat. Grill both sides for a few minutes on a hot greased grill or skillet until golden brown. Serve with margarine and honey or imitation maple syrup. Makes 6 slices.

Each slice equals: **1/2 OUNCE MEAT**
                                1 SALTED STARCH

Extra french toast can be placed on a cookie sheet, cooled and frozen for a few hours. After french toast is frozen, place it in a plastic bag. Thaw and heat individual slices in your toaster.

SPICED FRENCH TOAST

Add 1 teaspoon vanilla, 1/4 teaspoon nutmeg, and 1/4 teaspoon cinnamon to milk and egg mixture in french toast recipe above and proceed as directed.

DESSERTS

DESSERTS

DESSERTS

DESSERTS

2-CRUST PIE SHELL

2 Cups Sifted Flour
3/4 Cup Shortening
4 to 5 Tablespoons Ice Water

Cut shortening into flour until mixture resembles coarse cornmeal. Quickly sprinkle ice water, 1 tablespoon at a time, tossing lightly with a fork. (Pastry should be moist enough to hold together, not sticky). Shape pastry into a ball, cover and refrigerate until ready to use.

Divide pastry in half. Roll out to 11-inch circle and place in pan. Turn prepared filling into pan. Roll out top crust, make several gashes near center for steam vents, place on filling, crimp edges and bake as directed.

1-CRUST PIE SHELL

1 Cup Flour
1/3 Cup, Plus 1 Tablespoon Shortening
2 to 2-1/2 Tablespoons Ice Water

Follow directions for 2-crust pie shell above. Roll out to 11-inch circle and place in pan.

If pie and filling are not to be baked together, prick bottom and sides well with fork. Bake at 450° for 10 to 12 minutes or until golden.

GRAHAM CRACKER PIE SHELL

8 Large Graham Cracker Rectangles, Crushed
1/4 Cup Sugar
1/4 Cup Margarine, Melted

Combine crushed graham crackers, sugar and melted margarine. Pat into a 9-inch pie pan, evenly covering bottom and sides of pan. Chill for 1 hour or bake at 350° for 10 minutes and cool before filling.

APPLE CRUMB PIE

Pastry for 1-Crust Pie Shell
  (See recipe page E 1)
6 Cups Pared, Sliced, Tart Apples
1/2 Cup Sugar
1 Teaspoon Cinnamon
1/2 Cup Sugar
3/4 Cup Flour
1/3 Cup Margarine

Arrange apples in 9-inch pastry-lined pie pan. Mix 1/2 cup sugar with cinnamon; sprinkle over apples. Mix 1/2 cup sugar with flour, cut in margarine until crumbly. Sprinkle over apples. Bake at 400° for 40 to 50 minutes until apples are tender. Cut into 10 slices.

Each slice equals: **1 UNSALTED STARCH**
                    1/2 FRUIT
                    2 CALORIE BOOSTERS

OLD-FASHIONED APPLE PIE

Pastry for 2-Crust Pie
  (See recipe page E 1)
1 Cup Sugar
2 Tablespoons Flour
1 Teaspoon Cinnamon
1/8 Teaspoon Nutmeg
7 Cups Sliced Peeled Apples
2 Tablespoons Margarine

Combine sugar, flour, cinnamon and nutmeg. Mix lightly through apples. Heap apples in pastry-lined 9-inch pie pan. Dot apples with margarine. Adjust top crust and cut vents. Bake at 425° for 50 to 60 minutes, or until crust is browned and apples are tender. Cut into 10 slices.

Each slice equals: **1 UNSALTED STARCH**
                            1/2 FRUIT
                            2 CALORIE BOOSTERS

RED APPLE BERRY PIE

Pastry for 2-Crust Pie Shell
  (See recipe page E 1)
2 Cups Fresh or Frozen Cranberries
4 Cups Peeled, Sliced, Cooking Apples
1-1/2 Cups Sugar
1/4 Teaspoon Nutmeg (Optional)
1 Teaspoon Cinnamon (Optional)
2 Tablespoons Margarine

Prepare dough for crust. Roll out half the dough and fit into 9-inch pie pan. Chop cranberries coarsely. Add to apples. Add sugar, flour, nutmeg and cinnamon. Stir well to mix. Fill pie crust. Dot with margarine. Cover with top crust, vent and crimp edges. Bake 10 minutes at 450° and reduce heat to 375°. Bake until apples are tender and crust is well browned, 35 to 40 minutes longer. Makes 10 servings.

Each serving equals: **1 UNSALTED STARCH**
                                1/2 FRUIT
                                3 CALORIE BOOSTERS

BERRY PIE

Pastry for 2-Crust Pie Shell
  (See recipe page E 1)
4 Cups Fresh or Frozen, Thawed Blackberries,
  Raspberries or Blueberries
1 Tablespoon Lemon Juice
1 Cup Sugar
1/4 Teaspoon Cinnamon (Optional)
1/8 Teaspoon Nutmeg (Optional)
Dash Ground Cloves (Optional)
2 Tablespoons Margarine

Prepare crust as directed. Fit bottom crust into 9-inch pie pan. Place berries in large bowl, sprinkle with lemon juice. Combine flour, sugar and spices (if desired). Add to berries, toss lightly to mix. Turn berries into pastry-lined pie shell, dot with margarine. Cover with top crust, vent and crimp edges. Bake at 400° 45 to 50 minutes, or until juices start to bubble through steam vents and crust is golden. Cool or wire rack, serve slightly warm. Makes 10 servings.

Each serving equals: **1 UNSALTED STARCH**
                            1/2 FRUIT
                            2 CALORIE BOOSTERS

CHERRY RASPBERRY PIE

Pastry for 2-Crust Pie Shell
  (See recipe page E 1)
One 10-Ounce Package Frozen Raspberries,
  Thawed and Drained, Reserve Juice
1/2 Cup Sugar
3 Tablespoons Cornstarch
Red Food Coloring
One 16-Ounce can Pitted Red Tart Cherries, Drained,
  Reserve Syrup
1 Cup Reserved Raspberry and Cherry Juices, Combined

Prepare pastry for a 2-crust pie, line 9-inch pie plate with half the pastry. In a saucepan combine sugar and cornstarch; stir in reserved syrup, a few drops of red food coloring and cherries. Cook and stir over low heat until thick and clear; stir in raspberries. Pour fruit mixture into pastry-lined pie plate. Adjust top crust over filling, vent and crimp edges. Bake at 425° for 30 minutes. Cut into 10 pieces.

Each slice equals: **1 UNSALTED STARCH**
                          1/2 FRUIT
                          2 CALORIE BOOSTERS

PEAR PEPPERMINT PIE

**Graham Cracker Pie Crust
  (See recipe page E 2)
One 16-Ounce Can Pear Halves
1 Envelope Unflavored Gelatin
3-1/2 cups "Cool Whip"
2 Tablespoons Sugar
1 Teaspoon Vanilla Extract
1/8 Teaspoon Peppermint Extract
Few Drops Red Food Color
2 Ounces Peppermint Candy, Crushed**

Drain pears; reserve 1/4 cup syrup. Soften gelatin in 1/4 cup pear syrup; heat until gelatin dissolves. Combine "Cool Whip", sugar, vanilla, peppermint extract and food color. Beat until sugar dissolves. Gradually beat in gelatin mixture. Fold in 1/4 cup peppermint candy. Pour into prepared pie crust. Chill thoroughly. Arrange pear halves on pie, sprinkle with remaining peppermint candy. Makes 8 servings.

**Each serving equals: 1 SALTED STARCH
                          1/2 FRUIT
                          2 CALORIE BOOSTERS**

SOUR CREAM PINEAPPLE PIE

1-Crust Pie Shell, Baked
  (See recipe page E 1)
3/4 Cup Sugar
1/4 Cup Flour
2-1/2 Cups Crushed Pineapple,
  Undrained
1 Cup Sour Cream

1 Tablespoon Lemon Juice
2 Slightly Beaten Egg Yolks
2 Egg Whites
1/2 Teaspoon Vanilla
1/4 Teaspoon Cream of Tartar
4 Tablespoons Sugar

Combine 3/4 cup sugar and flour in a saucepan. Stir in pineapple, sour cream and lemon juice; mix well. Cook and stir until mixture thickens and bubbles; cook, stirring, 2 minutes. Remove from heat. Stir some of the hot mixture into the egg yolks; return to hot mixture, stirring constantly. Cook and stir 2 minutes more. Spoon into cooked pie shell. Make meringue: Beat egg whites with vanilla and cream of tartar until soft peaks form. Gradually add sugar, beating until stiff and glossy peaks form and the sugar is dissolved. Spread meringue over hot filling, sealing to edge of pastry. Bake at 350° for 12 to 15 minutes, or until meringue is golden. Cool before cutting. Makes 10 servings.

Each serving equals: 1 UNSALTED STARCH
                         1/2 FRUIT
                         2 CALORIE BOOSTERS

PUMPKIN PIE

Pastry for 1-Crust Pie
  (See recipe page E 1)
1 Egg
1 Cup Sugar
1-1/2 Cups Pumpkin
1/8 Teaspoon Cloves

1/2 Teaspoon Ginger
1/2 Teaspoon Nutmeg
1-1/2 Teaspoon Cinnamon
1 Tablespoon Cornstarch
1-1/2 Cups "Coffee Rich"

Prepare pastry and place in 9-inch pie pan as directed. Beat egg and sugar. Add pumpkin, cloves, ginger, nutmeg, cinnamon, "Coffee Rich" and cornstarch. Beat until thoroughly combined. Pour into pie shell. Bake at 375° for 60 minutes or until knife inserted halfway between the center and edge of pie comes out clean. Makes 8 servings.

Each serving equals: **1 UNSALTED STARCH**
                                   1 FRUIT
                                   2 CALORIE BOOSTERS

STRAWBERRY PIE

**Pastry for 1-Crust Pie, Baked
  (See recipe page E 1)
2 Tablespoons Sugar
1 Tablespoon Water
4 Cups Strawberries
1-1/2 Cups Sugar
1 Cup Boiling Water
3 Tablespoons Cornstarch
1/4 Cup Water
Several Drops Red Food Coloring**

Boil 2 tablespoons sugar and 1 tablespoon water for 3 minutes. Brush over hot baked pie shell. Return to oven for 2 minutes more, cool. Wash, hull and drain berries. (Set aside several for garnish.) Put 3 cups of berries in pie shell. Mash remaining berries, add with sugar to boiling water. Simmer 5 minutes. Rub through sieve. Mix cornstarch and water, add to cooked berry mixture and cook 5 minutes, until clear. Add food coloring. Remove from heat and beat hard 2 minutes. Pour over berries. Garnish with "Cool Whip" and remaining berries. Cut into 8 slices.

Each slice equals: **1 UNSALTED STARCH
1/2 FRUIT
2 CALORIE BOOSTERS**

STRAWBERRY CREAM CHEESE PIE

Graham Cracker Crust
  (See recipe page E 2)
2 Cups Fresh Strawberries, Hulled
1/4 Cup Sugar
One 8-Ounce Package Cream Cheese, Softened
1/2 Teaspoon Vanilla
2 Cups "Cool Whip"

Prepare graham cracker crust according to recipe, using 9-inch pie pan. Arrange whole strawberries (pointing up) in bottom of crust. Save several berries for garnish. Gradually add sugar to cream cheese in bowl, blending well. Add vanilla. Fold in "Cool Whip" and spoon into pie shell over berries. Chill at least 3 hours. Garnish with remaining berries. Makes 10 servings.

Each serving equals: **1 SALTED STARCH**
                              1/2 FRUIT
                              1 CALORIE BOOSTER

IMPOSSIBLE PUMPKIN PIE

2 Eggs
3/4 Cup Sugar
2 Cups "Coffee Rich"
1/4 Teaspoon Cloves
1/2 Teaspoon Ginger

1/4 Teaspoon Nutmeg
1 Teaspoon Cinnamon
1-1/2 Cups Pumpkin
1/2 Cup Biscuit Mix
   (See Recipe Page D 12)

Blend all ingredients in blender. Pour into greased 9-inch pie pan. Bake at 350° for 50 to 60 minutes. Let stand 15 minutes. Serve with "Cool Whip". Makes 8 servings.

Each serving equals: **1 SALTED STARCH**
                            1 FRUIT
                            1 CALORIE BOOSTER

IMPOSSIBLE COCONUT PIE

4 Eggs
1/2 Cup Flour
3/4 Cup Sugar
2 Cups "Coffee Rich"
1 Cup Coconut
1 Teaspoon Vanilla
1/2 Cup Margarine, Cut in Small Pieces

Blend all ingredients in blender for 1 minute. Pour into greased and floured 10-inch pie plate. Bake at 350° for 45 minutes. To check for doneness, insert a knife halfway between center and edge of pie. If done, knife will come out clean. Cut into 8 pieces.

Each slice equals: **1/2 OUNCE MEAT**
                                1/2 FRUIT
                                1 SALTED FAT
                                2 CALORIE BOOSTERS

LEMON MERINGUE PIE

Pastry for 1-Crust Pie
(See recipe page E 1)
6 Tablespoons Cornstarch
3 Tablespoons Flour
1-3/4 Cup Sugar
2 Cups Water

3 Egg Yolks, Slightly Beaten
1/2 Cup Lemon Juice
1 Tablespoon Lemon Peel
1 Tablespoon Margarine
3 Egg Whites
1/4 Teaspoon Cream of Tartar
1/2 Cup Sugar

Prepare pie crust as directed and place in 9-inch pie pan. Prick entire surface evenly with fork. Refrigerate 30 minutes. Bake at 450° for 8 to 10 minutes until golden brown. Cool completely before filling.

Combine cornstarch, flour and 1-3/4 cup sugar in medium saucepan, mix well. Gradually add water, stir until smooth. Cook over medium heat, bring to a boil, stirring constantly. Boil for 1 minute. Remove from heat. Stir some of the hot mixture into the egg yolks. Return to hot mixture and stir to blend. Cook 2 more minutes. Remove from heat; stir in lemon juice, lemon peel and margarine. Pour into pie shell.

Beat egg whites and cream of tartar until frothy. Gradually beat in sugar. Continue beating until stiff peaks form. Spread meringue over lemon filling, carefully, sealing to edge of crust. Bake at 400° for 7 to 9 minutes until browned. Let cool completely. Makes 10 servings.

Each serving equals: 1 UNSALTED STARCH
2 CALORIE BOOSTERS

UPSIDE-DOWN LEMON MERINGUE PIE

1 Tablespoon Shortening
2 Egg Whites
1/4 Teaspoon Cream of Tartar
1/2 Cup Sugar
2 Egg Yolks
1 Cup Sugar
1/4 Cup Cornstarch

1 Envelope Unflavored Gelatin
1 Cup Water
2 Tablespoons Margarine
1 Teaspoon Fresh Lemon Peel
1/3 Cup Fresh Lemon Juice
2 Cups "Cool Whip"
1-1/2 Cups "Cool Whip"

Grease a 9-inch pie plate with shortening. Beat egg whites and cream of tartar with an electric beater at high speed until soft peaks form. Add the 1/2 cup sugar, 1 tablespoon at a time, beating well after each addition. Beat until stiff peaks form. Spoon meringue into prepared pie plate, spread over bottom and up sides, forming a rim. Bake at 275° for 1 hour. Turn off heat and let meringue cool completely with oven door ajar. If desired, meringue can be removed from pie plate. (Meringue shell keeps well stored in an airtight container in a cool, dry place.)

Beat egg yolks in large bowl. In a medium-sized saucepan, mix 1 cup sugar, cornstarch and gelatin. Stir in water and cook over moderately high heat, stirring constantly, until gelatin dissolves completely and mixture is clear. Slowly add half the hot gelatin mixture to the egg yolks, stirring constantly. Return yolk mixture to the pan and cook 2 to 3 minutes over moderate heat, stirring constantly, until thickened slightly. Remove from heat, stir in margarine, lemon peel and juice. Pour mixture back into bowl and refrigerate 8 to 12 minutes, until consistancy of unbeaten egg whites. Fold in 2 cups of "Cool Whip" and pour mixture into meringue shell. Spread remaining 1-1/2 cups "Cool Whip" over filling. Refrigerate 4 hours or more, until filling is set. Makes 8 servings.

Each serving equals: 1 UNSALTED STARCH
2 CALORIE BOOSTERS

SOUTHERN PECAN PIE

Pastry for 1-Crust Pie Shell
  (See Recipe Page E 1)
1-1/4 Cups Water
1-1/4 Cups Sugar
1/4 Cup Margarine
3/4 Cup Sugar
3 Egg Yolks
1/4 Cup Flour
1 Teaspoon Vanilla
1 Cup Pecan Halves*

Prepare pastry and place in 9-inch pie pan, as directed. Set aside. Prepare syrup by boiling water and 1-1/4 cups sugar over medium-high heat for 15 minutes. Cream margarine. Add 3/4 cup sugar gradually, creaming after each addition. Add 1 cup of syrup, egg yolks and flour. Mix thoroughly. Stir in vanilla and pecans. Pour into prepared pie shell. Bake at 350° for about 1 hour or until set. Cool. Cut into 10 slices.

Each slice equals: **1 UNSALTED STARCH**
                           1/2 FRUIT
                           3 CALORIE BOOSTERS

* Pecans are high in potassium. They have been specially
  calculated into this recipe. Use only as directed.

ANGEL PIE

Graham Cracker Crust
  (See Recipe Page E 2)
4 Cups Packed Marshmallows
1/2 Cup Milk
2 Cups "Cool Whip"
1/2 Teaspoon Almond Extract
One 17-Ounce Can Fruit Cocktail, Drained

Prepare graham cracker crust as directed using 9-inch pie pan. Melt marshmallows in milk in top of double boiler; set aside to cool. Combine "Cool Whip", almond extract and fruit cocktail; fold in cooled marshmallow mixture. Pour into graham cracker crust and refrigerate 8 hours or more. Cut into 8 slices.

Each slice equals: **1 SALTED STARCH**
                            1 FRUIT
                            2 CALORIE BOOSTERS

LIGHT AND FRUITY PIE

Graham Cracker Crust
  (See Recipe Page E 2)
One 3-Ounce Package Flavored Gelatin
2/3 Cup Boiling Water
2 Cups Ice Cubes
One 8-Ounce Container "Cool Whip"
1 Cup Fruit (Use 1 Cup Diced Fresh Strawberries, Blueberries or
  Raspberries or Canned, Drained, Crushed Pineapple

Prepare graham cracker crust in 9-inch pie pan as directed. Dissolve gelatin in boiling water, stirring constantly about 3 minutes. Add ice cubes and stir until gelatin is thickened, about 2 to 3 minutes. Remove any unmelted ice. Blend in "Cool Whip" stir until smooth. Fold in fruit. Chill until mixture mounds. Spoon into pie crust. Chill 3 hours. Cut into 8 pieces.

Each serving equals: **1 SALTED STARCH**
                              1/2 FRUIT
                              1 CALORIE BOOSTER

BRANDY ALEXANDER PIE

1/4 Cup Margarine
1-1/2 Cups Vanilla Wafer Crumbs
3 Cups Miniature Marshmallows, Packed
1/2 Cup Milk
1/4 Cup Dark Creme de Cocoa
1/4 Cup Cognac
2 Cups "Cool Whip"
1 Ounce Semi-Sweet Chocolate

Melt margarine and stir in cookie crumbs. Press mixture firmly and evenly over bottom and up sides of a 9-inch pie pan. Bake at 350° for 10 minutes. Remove from oven and let cool completely. In a medium sized saucepan, heat marshmallows and milk over low heat, stirring constantly, until marshmallows are melted. Remove from heat and stir until smooth. Beat in creme de cocoa and cognac, using a wire whisk or rotary beater. When well mixed, chill 20 to 30 minutes, stirring once or twice, until mixture mounds slightly when dropped from a spoon. Fold "Cool Whip" into marshmallow mixture. Pour into pie shell, cover and chill 4 hours or more. Shortly before serving, "peel" chocolate with a vegetable peeler and let the curls fall on the top of the pie. Makes 8 servings.

Each serving equals: **1 SALTED STARCH**
                             3 CALORIE BOOSTERS

GRASSHOPPER PIE

Substitute green creme de menthe and clear creme de cocoa for cognac and dark creme de cocoa.

SWEET CHOCOLATE CREAM PIE

Graham Cracker Crust (See Recipe Page E 2)
4 Ounces Sweet Chocolate
1/3 Cup Milk
2 Tablespoons Sugar
One 3-Ounce Package Cream Cheese, Softened
2 Cups "Cool Whip"

Prepare graham cracker crust; set aside. Make several chocolate curls from chocolate with sharp knife; set aside for garnish. Heat chocolate and 2 tablespoons milk over low heat, stirring until melted. Beat sugar into cream cheese; add remaining milk and chocolate mixture. Beat until smooth. Fold "Cool Whip" into chocolate mixture. Blend until smooth. Spoon mixture into crust. Freeze about 4 hours. Garnish with chocolate curls. Makes 10 servings.

Each serving equals: **1 UNSALTED STARCH**
                             1/2 FRUIT
                             1 CALORIE BOOSTER

COFFEE CLOUD PIE

1 Graham Cracker Pie Shell (See Recipe Page E 2)
4 Cups Marshmallows, Packed
2 Teaspoons Instant Coffee
1 Cup Water
1 Tablespoon Margarine
1 Tablespoon Brandy
2 Cups "Cool Whip"

Prepare pie shell according to recipe; set aside. Combine marshmallows, coffee, water and margarine in top of double boiler. Heat until marshmallows melt. Add brandy. Remove from heat and refrigerate 20 to 30 minutes until mixture starts to thicken. Fold in "Cool Whip" and heap into pie shell. Refrigerate. Makes 8 servings.

Each serving equals: **1 SALTED STARCH**
                           2 CALORIE BOOSTERS

FROZEN MINT PIE

1-1/2 Cups Crushed Chocolate Wafers
1/3 Cup Margarine, Melted
Mint Bavarian (See Recipe Page E 46)
"Cool Whip"

Combine crushed chocolate wafers and melted margarine. Pat into 9-inch pie pan, covering sides and bottom evenly. Bake at 350° for 10 minutes. Cool. Make mint bavarian following the recipe. Spoon into chocolate wafer pie shell and freeze. Serve frozen, garnished with "Cool Whip". Makes 6 servings.

Each serving equals: **1/2 SALTED STARCH**
1 SALTED FAT
2 CALORIE BOOSTERS

APPLESAUCE LOAF CAKE

1/4 Cup Margarine
1/2 Cup Brown Sugar*
1/2 Cup Sugar
1 Teaspoon Cinnamon
1/2 Teaspoon Cloves
1/4 Teaspoon Nutmeg
2 Cups Flour
1 Cup Applesauce
1 Teaspoon Baking Soda
1 Cup Raisins

GLAZE:
1 Cup Confectioners' Sugar
1-1/2 Tablespoons Lemon Juice

Cream margarine, add brown sugar, sugar, cinnamon, cloves and nutmeg. Beat until well blended. Stir in flour, applesauce and baking soda; beat well. Add raisins and pour into lightly greased loaf pan. Bake at 350° for 60 to 70 minutes or until done. Let stand in pan 10 minutes before removing. Place on wire rack, drizzle with glaze made of confectioners' sugar and lemon juice. Cut into 10 slices.

Each slice equals: **1 SALTED STARCH**
                            1 FRUIT
                            2 CALORIE BOOSTERS

* Brown sugar is high in potassium. It has been specially calculated into this recipe. Use it only as directed.

BROWN MOUNTAIN CAKE

1 Cup Milk
1 Tablespoon Lemon Juice
1 Cup Margarine
2 Cups Sugar
3 Eggs
3 Cups Flour

1 Teaspoon Baking Soda
3 Tablespoons Unsweetened
  Cocoa
1 Teaspoon Vanilla
1/2 Cup Warm Water

Combine milk and lemon juice. Let stand. Cream margarine and sugar; beat in eggs one at a time. Mix flour, baking soda and cocoa; add alternately with milk to creamed mixture. Stir in vanilla and warm water. Pour into 9 x 13-inch greased and floured pan. Bake at 350° for 45 minutes. Cool and frost. Cut into 24 pieces.

Each piece equals: **1 SALTED STARCH**
                           1 CALORIE BOOSTER

CRANBERRY UPSIDE-DOWN CAKE

3 Tablespoons Margarine, Softened
1/2 Cup Sugar
1 Pound Fresh Cranberries (Rinsed, Picked-Over,
  Patted Dry)
6 Tablespoons Margarine, Softened
1/2 Cup Sugar
1 Egg
1 Teaspoon Vanilla
1 Teaspoon Orange Rind
1-1/4 Cup Flour
1-1/2 Teaspoon Baking Powder
1/3 Cup Red Currant Jelly

Grease bottom and sides of 9-inch cake pan with 3 tablespoons margarine. Sprinkle 1/2 cup sugar evenly over bottom, top with cranberries. Cream margarine, sugar and egg. Add vanilla and orange rind, beat well. Set aside. In another bowl, mix flour and baking powder. Stir the flour mixture into the sugar mixture, 1/2 cup at a time, alternately with milk. Stir just until combined. Pour the batter over the cranberries, smooth the top and bake on a cookie sheet in the center of a preheated 350° oven for 1 hour or until well browned. Transfer the cake to a rack and let it cool 20 minutes. Run a thin knife around the inside of the pan and invert onto serving plate. In a small saucepan melt jelly over low heat, stirring. Brush melted jelly over cake. Serve warm or at room temperature, topped with "Cool Whip", if desired. Makes 12 servings.

Each serving equals: **1 SALTED STARCH**
                                       1 CALORIE BOOSTER

EASY LAYER CAKE

2 Cups Sifted Cake Flour*   1 Cup Milk
1 Cup Sugar   1 Egg
2-1/2 Teaspoons Baking Powder   1 Teaspoon Vanilla
1/3 Cup Margarine

Mix flour, sugar and baking powder. Add margarine and milk; beat at medium speed with electric mixer for 2 minutes. Add egg and vanilla, beat 2 minutes more. Pour into 2 greased and floured 9-inch cake pans. Bake at 350° for 25 to 30 minutes. Cool in pans 10 minutes. Remove cake from pans and cool thoroughly on wire rack and frost. Cut into 16 pieces.

Each piece equals: 1 SALTED STARCH

* 1-3/4 cup sifted all-purpose flour may be
  substituted for sifted cake flour.

JELLY-ROLL CAKE

4 Eggs
3/4 Cup Sifted Cake Flour
1 Teaspoon Baking Powder
3/4 Cup Sugar

Confectioners' Sugar
1 Cup Raspberry Preserves

In small bowl, let eggs warm to room temperature, about 1 hour. Lightly grease bottom of 15 x 10 x 1-inch jelly-roll pan; then line bottom with waxed paper. Mix flour and baking powder, set aside. At high speed, beat eggs until very thick and lemon colored. Beat in granulated sugar, 2 tablespoons at a time; continue beating 5 more minutes, or until very thick. Gently fold in flour mixture, just until combined. Turn into prepared pan, spreading evenly. Bake at 400° for 9 minutes or just until surface springs back when gently pressed with fingertip.

Meanwhile, on a clean tea towel, sift confectioners' sugar, forming a 15 x 10-inch rectangle. Invert cake on sugar; gently peel off waxed paper. Starting with narrow end, roll up cake (towel and all). Place, seam side down, on wire rack to cool, about 20 minutes. Gently unroll cake, remove towel. Spread with preserves; roll up again. Place seam side down on serving plate; let stand covered at least 1 hour before serving. To serve, sift confectioners' sugar over top; slice on diagonal. Serve with a bowl of "Cool Whip", if desired. Makes 16 servings.

Each serving equals: 1 UNSALTED STARCH

* 2/3 cup sifted all-purpose flour may be substituted
  for sifted cake flour.

KNOBBY APPLE CAKE

3 Tablespoons Margarine
1/4 Cup Sugar
3/4 Cup Honey
1 Egg
2 Cups Flour
1 Teaspoon Baking Powder

1/2 Teaspoon Baking Soda
1/4 Teaspoon Nutmeg
1 Teaspoon Lemon Extract
3 Cups Diced, Peeled
   Cooking Apples

Cream margarine and sugar, add honey, beat well. Add egg and mix. Add flour, baking power, baking soda and nutmeg; mix well. Add lemon extract and apples, pour into 9-inch square pan. Bake at 350° for 55 to 60 minutes. Serve warm with lemon nutmeg sauce.

HOT LEMON NUTMEG SAUCE

1 Tablespoon Cornstarch
1/2 Cup Sugar
2 Tablespoons Grated Lemon Rind
1 Cup Water
1/4 Cup Lemon Juice
2 Tablespoons Margarine
Dash Nutmeg

Mix cornstarch, sugar and lemon rind. Add water and cook 5 minutes until thick. Remove from heat, add lemon juice, margarine and nutmeg. Makes 12 servings.

Each serving equals: 1 UNSALTED STARCH
                         1/2 FRUIT
                         1 CALORIE BOOSTER

MARBLE LOAF CAKE

1-1/2 Squares Unsweetened Chocolate
2-1/2 Cups Sifted Cake Flour*
3 Teaspoons Baking Powder
1/2 Cup Margarine
1-1/2 Cups Sugar
3 Eggs
3/4 Teaspoon Vanilla
3/4 Cup Milk

Melt chocolate over hot, not boiling water. Let cool. Preheat oven to 350°. Grease and flour a 9 x 5-inch loaf pan (or two 8-inch layer pans). Mix flour and baking powder. Set aside. Beat margarine and sugar until light, add eggs and vanilla, beating until very light and fluffy. Beat in flour mixture (in fourths), alternately with milk (in thirds), beginning and ending with flour mixture. In a medium bowl, combine about one-third batter with chocolate, mixing well. Spoon plain and chocolate batters, alternately, into prepared pan. With knife cut through batter, forming a Z to marbleize. Bake 65 minutes for loaf pan, 30-35 minutes for layer pans, until done. Cool in pan 15 minutes, remove and cool thoroughly on wire racks. Frost. Cut into 24 slices.

Each slice equals:　　　**1 SALTED STARCH**

*2 cups plus 3 tablespoons sifted all-purpose flour may be substituted for sifted cake flour.

PINEAPPLE UPSIDE-DOWN CAKE

1/4 Cup Margarine
1/2 Cup Brown Sugar*
One 17-1/2-Ounce Can Sliced Pineapple, Drained
5 Maraschino Cherries
1/2 Cup Margarine
3/4 Cup Sugar
1 Teaspoon Vanilla
1-3/4 Cups Sifted Cake Flour
   (or 1-1/2 Cups Sifted All-Purpose Flour)
2 Teaspoons Baking Powder
3/4 Cup Ice Water
2 Egg Whites
1/4 Cup Sugar

Melt 1/4 cup margarine in 9-inch round pan. Sprinkle with brown sugar. Arrange pineapple and cherries in pan. Cream 1/2 cup margarine with 3/4 cup sugar; add vanilla. Sift together flour and baking powder, add to margarine mixture alternately with ice water; beat well after each addition. Beat egg whites until foamy, gradually add 1/4 cup sugar and beat until stiff peaks form. Fold in batter. Pour over pineapple and brown sugar mixture in pan. Bake at 350° for 50 to 55 minutes, or until done. Invert cake on serving dish to cool. Makes 9 servings.

Each serving equals: 1 SALTED STARCH
                           1/2 FRUIT
                           1 SALTED FAT
                           1 CALORIE BOOSTER

*Brown sugar is high in potassium. It has been specially calculated into this recipe. Use it only as directed.

TEXAS CAKE

CAKE:
- 1 Cup Water
- 1 Cup Margarine
- 1/4 Cup Unsweetened Cocoa
- 2 Cups Flour
- 2 Cups Sugar
- 1 Teaspoon Baking Soda
- 2 Eggs
- 1/2 Cup Sour Cream

FROSTING:
- 1/2 Cup Margarine
- 6 Tablespoons Milk
- 3 Tablespoons Unsweetened Cocoa
- 3-1/2 Cups Confectioners' Sugar
- 1 Tablespoon Vanilla

Heat water, margarine and cocoa until margarine is melted. Mix flour, sugar, baking soda, eggs and sour cream into cocoa mixture. Pour into ungreased 15 x 10 x 1-inch jelly-roll pan (batter is thin.) Bake at 350° for 20 minutes.

FROSTING: Heat margarine, milk and cocoa until margarine is melted. Mix in confectioners' sugar and vanilla. Pour hot frosting over hot cake. Makes 24 servings.

Each serving equals: 1 SALTED STARCH
1 CALORIE BOOSTER

WESTERN GINGERBREAD

1 Cup Milk
1 Tablespoon Lemon Juice
2 Cups Flour
1-1/4 Cup Sugar
1 Teaspoon Baking Powder
1 Teaspoon Cinnamon

1-1/2 Teaspoon Ginger
1/2 Cup Margarine
1 Egg
2 Tablespoons Molasses*
1 Teaspoon Baking Soda
1 Tablespoon Margarine

Mix milk and lemon juice. Let stand. Mix flour, sugar, baking powder, cinnamon and ginger. Cut in 1/2 cup margarine until fine. Reserve 1/2 cup of crumb mixture for topping. Add baking soda to milk mixture and dissolve. To remaining crumbs, add egg, molasses and milk mixture. Beat with electric mixer for 2 minutes on low speed. Pour into greased 13 x 9-inch pan. Cut 1 tablespoon margarine into reserved crumb mixture. Sprinkle over batter. Bake at 350° for 30-35 minutes. Cut into 18 pieces.

Each piece equals: **1 SALTED STARCH**
                            1 CALORIE BOOSTER

* Molasses is high in potassium. It has been specially calculated in this recipe. Use only as directed.

BANANA SPLIT DESSERT

6 Whole Graham Crackers, Crushed
2 Tablespoon Margarine, Melted
1 Egg
1/4 Cup Margarine
1 Cup Confectioners' Sugar
1 Cup Undrained, Crushed Pineapple
1 Medium Banana, Thinly Sliced
2 Cups "Cool Whip"

Combine graham cracker crumbs and margarine. Pat into an 8-inch square pan. Set aside. Combine egg, margarine and confectioners' sugar; beat for 15 minutes. Pour over crust. Top with crushed pineapple and banana slices. Spread "Cool Whip" on top. Makes 9 servings.

Each serving equals: **1 SALTED STARCH**
                              1/2 FRUIT
                              1 CALORIE BOOSTER

QUICK CHEESECAKE DESSERT

Graham Cracker Crust (See Recipe Page E 2)
FILLING:
  8 Ounces Cream Cheese, Softened
  1/2 Cup Powdered Sugar
  2 Cups "Cool Whip"

Combine crust ingredients, pat into 8-inch square pan. Combine cream cheese, powdered sugar and "Cool Whip"; beat with electric mixer on high until light and fluffy. Spoon into crust. Top with one of the following fruit glazes. Cut into 8 servings.

Each serving equals: **1 SALTED STARCH**
                              1 FRUIT
                              1 SALTED FAT
                              1 CALORIE BOOSTER

RED CHERRY GLAZE

One 16-Ounce Can Tart Red Cherries,
  Drained, Reserve 1/2 Cup Liquid
1/4 Cup Sugar
1 Tablespoon Cornstarch
1 Tablespoon Lemon Juice
2 Drops Red Food Coloring

In small saucepan, combine sugar and cornstarch. Add reserved cherry liquid, stirring until mixture is smooth. Bring to boiling and boil 2 to 3 minutes until thick and clear. Remove from heat, cool slightly. Add lemon juice, cherries and food coloring. Cool thoroughly before spooning over dessert.

See page E 36 for other glazes.

STRAWBERRY OR BLUEBERRY GLAZE

**One 10-Ounce Package Frozen Halved Strawberries
  or Blueberries, Thawed
1 Tablespoon Sugar
2 Teaspoons Cornstarch**

Drain the berries, reserving 1/2 cup of the liquid (add water if necessary). In a small saucepan, combine sugar and cornstarch. Stir in reserved liquid. Over medium heat, bring to boiling and boil, stirring, 1 minute. Remove from heat; cool slightly. Stir in berries and cool completely before spooning over dessert.

PINEAPPLE GLAZE

**1 Tablespoon Sugar
2 Teaspoons Cornstarch
1 Cup Crushed Pineapple, Undrained**

In small saucepan, combine sugar and cornstarch. Stir in pineapple. Over medium heat, bring to boiling, stirring, boil 1 minute. Cool completely before spooning over dessert.

FROZEN CHOCOLATE CHIP CHEESECAKE

1-1/4 Cups Crushed Graham Crackers (16 Squares)
1/4 Cup Sugar
6 Tablespoons Margarine, Melted
One 8-Ounce Package
  Plus One 3-Ounce Package Cream Cheese, Softened
1 Quart Chocolate Ice Cream
1/2 Cup Semisweet Chocolate Chips, Chopped

Combine graham cracker crumbs, sugar and margarine. Press on the bottom and 1-3/4-inches up the sides of an 8-inch spring-form pan. Chill. Beat cream cheese with electric mixer, until fluffy. Set aside. Stir ice cream just enough to soften, gradually add to cream cheese, beating with mixer until smooth. Fold in chopped chocolate chips (save a tablespoon for garnish). Pour into crust. Cover and freeze 8 hours or overnight. To serve, let stand at room temperature 30 to 40 minutes. Garnish with "Cool Whip," if desired, and reserved chocolate. Makes 10 servings.

Each serving equals: **1 MILK**
                             1 SALTED STARCH
                             2 CALORIE BOOSTERS

TROPICAL CHEESECAKE

1/2 Cup Graham Cracker Crumbs
2 Tablespoons Margarine, Melted
One 8-Ounce Package Cream Cheese, Softened
1/2 Cup Sifted Confectioners' Sugar
2-1/2 Cups Crushed Pineapple, Well Drained
2 Cups "Cool Whip"

Mix graham cracker crumbs and margarine, reserve 2 tablespoons for garnish. Press crumbs on the bottom of an 8-inch round cake pan; chill. Whip cream cheese and confectioners' sugar until fluffy. Stir in pineapple and "Cool Whip". Spread over crust. Sprinkle with reserved crumbs; chill well. Makes 8 servings.

Each serving equals: **1 SALTED STARCH**
                            1/2 FRUIT
                            1 CALORIE BOOSTER

BREAD PUDDING

2 Cups "Coffee Rich"
1/2 Cup Sugar
2 Eggs, Beaten
1 Teaspoon Vanilla
1/2 Teaspoon Cinnamon
2 Cups Bread Cubes
1/2 Cup Raisins* (Optional)

Combine "Coffee Rich", sugar, eggs, vanilla and cinnamon in a large bowl. Stir in bread cubes and raisins. Pour into 1-quart baking dish. Set in pan of hot water about 1-inch deep. Bake at 350° for 50 minutes, or until knife inserted in center of custard comes out clean. Makes 4 servings.

Each serving equals: 1/2 OUNCE MEAT
                                 1/2 SALTED STARCH
                                 1 FRUIT*
                                 3 CALORIE BOOSTERS

*If raisins are omitted from this recipe count each serving as:
                                 1/2 OUNCE MEAT
                                 1/2 SALTED STARCH
                                 3 CALORIE BOOSTERS

BROWNIE PUDDING

1 Cup Flour	1 Teaspoon Vanilla
2 Teaspoons Baking Powder	2 Tablespoons Margarine, Melted
3/4 Cup Sugar	3/4 Cup Brown Sugar*
2 Tablespoons Unsweetened Cocoa*	1/4 Cup Unsweetened Cocoa*
1/2 Cup Milk	1-3/4 Cup Hot Water

Mix flour, baking powder, sugar and 2 tablespoons cocoa. Add milk, vanilla and melted margarine; mix until smooth. Pour into 8 x 8-inch pan. Mix brown sugar and 1/4 cup cocoa, sprinkle over batter. Carefully pour hot water over batter. Bake at 350° for 40-45 minutes. Serve warm. Makes 8 servings.

Each serving equals: 1 SALTED STARCH
1 FRUIT
1 CALORIE BOOSTER

* The cocoa and brown sugar raise the potassium content of this recipe so that a serving of fruit must be counted for each serving.

FESTIVE CRANBERRY TORTE

Graham Cracker Crust (See Recipe Page E 2)
2 Cups Fresh Cranberries
1 Cup Sugar
2 Egg Whites
1 Teaspoon Orange Extract
1 Teaspoon Vanilla
2 Cups "Cool Whip"
1/2 Cup Sugar
1 Tablespoon Cornstarch
3/4 Cup Fresh Cranberries
2/3 Cup Water

Prepare graham cracker crust, press into the bottom and up sides of an 8-inch springform pan. Chill. Coarsely grind 2 cups of fresh cranberries, combine with 1 cup sugar and let stand 5 minutes. Add unbeaten egg whites, orange extract and vanilla Beat on low speed of electric mixer until frothy. Then beat at high speed 6 to 8 minutes or until stiff peaks form. Fold "Cool Whip" into cranberry mixture. Turn into crust and freeze until firm.

Prepare cranberry glaze. Stir 1/2 cup sugar and cornstarch together in a saucepan; stir in 3/4 cup whole cranberries and water. Cook stirring occasionally, just until cranberry skins pop. Cool to room temperature (do not chill). To serve. Remove torte from pan. Place on serving plate. Spoon cranberry glaze in center. Makes 8 servings.

Each serving equals: **1 UNSALTED STARCH**
                               2 CALORIE BOOSTERS

GLORIFIED RICE

3-1/2 Cups "Cool Whip"
1/2 Teaspoon Vanilla
2 Cups Cooked Rice
2/3 Cup Drained Crushed Pineapple
1 Cup Miniature Marshmallows

Blend vanilla into "Cool Whip". Combine rice, pineapple and marshmallows, fold into "Cool Whip" and chill. Makes eight 3/4-cup servings.

Each serving equals: 1/2 UNSALTED STARCH
                        1 CALORIE BOOSTER

LEMON PUDDING

1/2 Cup Lemon Juice   1-1/2 Tablespoons Cornstarch
1 Cup Water   1/3 Cup Water
1/2 Cup Sugar   4 Tablespoons Margarine
2 Drops Yellow Food Coloring 1 Teaspoon Lemon Peel

Combine lemon juice with 1 cup water and sugar in a saucepan, bring to a boil. Add food coloring. Mix cornstarch with 1/3 cup water, add to lemon mixture all at once. Cook 2 minutes stirring constantly. Remove from heat. Add margarine and lemon peel, beat until thoroughly mixed. Pour into 4 individual dishes and cool. Makes 4 servings.

Each serving equals: 1 SALTED FAT
                        1 CALORIE BOOSTER

RICE CUSTARD

2 Cups "Coffee Rich"
1/3 Cup Sugar
2 Tablespoons Margarine
2 Eggs, Beaten
1 Cup Cooked Rice
1/2 Cup Raisins
1 Teaspoon Vanilla

Heat "Coffee Rich" till steaming; add sugar and margarine. And mixture slowly to eggs, stirring constantly. Stir in rice, raisins, and vanilla. Pour into 1-quart baking dish. Set in a pan of hot water about 1-inch deep. Bake at 350° for 30-40 minutes, or until knife inserted in center of custard comes out clean. Makes four 3/4-cup servings.

Each serving equals: 1/2 OUNCE MEAT
                       1/2 UNSALTED STARCH
                       1 FRUIT
                       1 SALTED FAT
                       2 CALORIE BOOSTERS

NOTE: 1/4 teaspoon cinnamon and nutmeg may be added to rice custard with vanilla if desired.

LEMON BAVARIAN

2 Tablespoons Cornstarch
1/4 Cup Water
1/2 Cup Sugar
3/4 Cup Water
1/4 Cup Frozen Concentrated Lemonade
2 Drops Yellow Food Coloring
1 Tablespoon Margarine
2 Cups "Cool Whip"

Mix cornstarch and 1/4 cup water in small saucepan. Stir in sugar and 3/4 cup water. Cook over medium heat, stirring constantly, until mixture thickens and begins to boil. Boil and stir 1 minute. Remove from heat; stir in frozen concentrated lemonade, food coloring and margarine. Press plastic wrap on top of bavarian to prevent skin from forming, refrigerate just until cool. Fold in "Cool Whip". Refrigerate or freeze for a frozen dessert. Makes six 1/2-cup servings.

Each serving equals: 2 CALORIE BOOSTERS

LIME BAVARIAN

Follow directions for lemon bavarian substituting frozen concentrated limeade and green food coloring for lemonade and yellow food coloring.

LIME SNOW

2 Envelopes Unflavored Gelatin
1 Cup Cold Water
1/4 Cup Sugar
One 6-Ounce Can Frozen Limeade Concentrate (Keep Frozen)
1/2 Cup Ice Water
2 Egg Whites

Sprinkle gelatin over cold water in saucepan. Place over low heat; stir constantly until gelatin dissolves, 2 to 3 minutes. Stir in sugar, stir to dissolve. Remove from heat. Add limeade concentrate and ice water; stir until melted. Chill until slightly thicker than consistency of unbeaten egg white. Add egg whites to gelatin mixture, beat until mixture begins to hold its shape. Turn into 6-cup mold. Chill until firm. Unmold; garnish and serve with "Cool Whip". Makes eight 1/2-cup servings.

Each serving equals: 1 UNSALTED STARCH

MINT BAVARIAN

2 Tablespoons Cornstarch
1/4 Cup Water
1/2 Cup Sugar
3/4 Cup Water
1 Teaspoon Peppermint Extract
1 Tablespoon Margarine
Few Drops Green or Red Food Coloring
2 Cups "Cool Whip"

Mix cornstarch and 1/4 cup water in small saucepan. Stir in sugar and 3/4 cup water. Cook over medium heat, stirring constantly, until mixture thickens and begins to boil. Boil and stir 1 minute. Remove from heat; stir in extract, margarine and food coloring. Press plastic wrap on top of bavarian to prevent skin from forming, refrigerate just until cool. Fold in "Cool Whip". Refrigerate or freeze for a frozen dessert. Makes six 1/2-cup servings.

Each serving equals: 2 CALORIE BOOSTERS

STRAWBERRY BAVARIAN CREAM

**Three 10-Ounce Packages Sweetened
  Frozen Strawberries, Thawed
1 Tablespoon Lemon Juice
2 Envelopes Unflavored Gelatin
1/2 Cup Sugar
1 Egg
1 Cup Heavy Cream
1 Cup Crushed Ice
2 Tablespoons Cognac or Orange Flavored
  Liquor (Optional)**

Drain 2 packages of strawberries, save juice. Save remaining package to serve over bavarian. Measure 1/2 cup drained strawberry juice into saucepan and add lemon juice. Heat to simmering. Soften gelatin in 1/4 cup cold strawberry juice. Pour hot strawberry juice into blendor, add gelatin mixture, cover and blend 45 seconds. Add the drained strawberries, sugar and egg. Cover and blend 5 seconds at high speed. Add cream and ice, cover and blend 25 seconds. Pour into a 1-1/2-quart mold rinsed with cold water. Chill at least 2 hours. Mix remaining package of strawberries with cognac. Unmold bavarian and serve with strawberry sauce. Makes 8 servings.

**Each serving equals: 1 UNSALTED STARCH
                             1 FRUIT
                             1 CALORIE BOOSTER**

STRAWBERRY PARFAIT

4 Cups Strawberries, Washed, Hulled and Sliced
1/2 Cup Sugar
1/4 Cup Water
2 Egg Yolks
1 Tablespoon Lemon Juice
2 Cups "Cool Whip"
1/4 Cup Sugar

Crush 2 cups strawberries well and set aside. Mix 1/2 cup sugar and water in a saucepan. Bring to a boil and simmer 5 minutes. Beat egg yolks in top of double boiler; gradually stir in sugar syrup. Cook over simmering water, stirring constantly, until thick and lemon colored. Remove from heat. Continue beating until cool. Add crushed berries, lemon juice and "Cool Whip". Pour into refrigerator tray; freeze until firm. Serve with remaining strawberries sweetened with 1/4 cup sugar. Makes six 1-cup servings.

Each serving equals: 1 FRUIT
1 CALORIE BOOSTER

APPLE DUMPLINGS

1 Cup Sugar
1 Cup Water
1/4 Teaspoon Cinnamon
1/4 Teaspoon Nutmeg
4 to 6 Drops Red Food Coloring
2 Tablespoons Margarine
1-1/3 Cups Flour
1-1/2 Teaspoons Baking Powder

1/2 Cup Shortening
1/3 Cup Milk
4 Peeled, Pared Apples,
  Cut in Half
1/3 Cup Sugar
1/4 Teaspoon Cinnamon
1/4 Teaspoon Nutmeg
2 Tablespoons Margarine

To make syrup, combine 1 cup sugar, water, 1/4 teaspoon cinnamon, 1/4 teaspoon nutmeg, red food coloring and 2 tablespoons margarine in a small saucepan. Heat to boiling, boil 2 minutes and remove from heat.

Mix flour and baking powder, cut in shortening until mixture resembles coarse cornmeal, add milk and mix. Roll dough out on lightly floured surface into an 8 x 16-inch rectangle. Cut into eight 4-inch squares. Place an apple half on each square. Mix 1/3 cup sugar, 1/4 teaspoon cinnamon and 1/4 teaspoon nutmeg together; sprinkle on apples. Dot with 2 tablespoons of margarine. Pinch 4 corners of each square together at top of apple, pinch edges closed. Place apples in an 8 x 10-inch baking dish. Pour syrup gently over apples. Bake at 375° for 35 to 40 minutes until dumplings are golden and apples tender. Serve warm or cold. Makes 8 servings.

Each serving equals: 1 SALTED STARCH
                              1/2 FRUIT
                              3 CALORIE BOOSTERS

APPLE NUT COBBLER

4 Cups Tart, Thinly Sliced Apples
1/2 Cup Sugar
1/2 Teaspoon Cinnamon
1/2 Cup Pecans, Chopped*
1/2 Cup Margarine, Softened
1/2 Cup Sugar
1 Egg
3/4 Cup Flour
1/2 Teaspoon Vanilla

Slice apples into 10-inch pie plate. Sprinkle with mixture of 1/2 cup sugar and cinnamon. Top with chopped pecans. Cream margarine, gradually add 1/2 cup sugar, beating well. Stir in egg and beat well. Stir in flour and vanilla. Spread batter over apples. Bake at 375° for 35 minutes, until crisp and golden. Cut into 8 slices. Serve warm with "Cool Whip".

Each slice equals: **1 SALTED STARCH**
                            1 FRUIT
                            2 CALORIE BOOSTERS

* Nuts are high in potassium. They have been specially calculated into this recipe. Use only as directed.

BAKED APPLES

6 Large Apples
1 Cup Sugar
3 Tablespoons Orange Peel
1/2 Teaspoon Cinnamon
3 Tablespoons Margarine
1 Cup Boiling Water

Wash and core apples. Place in baking dish. Combine sugar, orange peel and cinnamon. Fill center of each apple with sugar mixture. Dot each apple with margarine. Pour boiling water into baking dish. Bake uncovered, at 375° until tender, about 1 hour; baste apples occasionally. Serve warm or cold. Makes 6 servings.

Each apple equals: 1 FRUIT
1/2 SALTED FAT
2 CALORIE BOOSTERS

BAKED SPICED PEACHES

6 Canned Peach Halves
2/3 Cup Syrup from Peaches
1/2 Cup Sugar
3 Tablespoons Margarine
2 Tablespoons Lemon Juice
3 Sticks Cinnamon
8 Whole Cloves

Arrange peach halves in a 1-1/2-quart casserole. In a saucepan, combine peach syrup, sugar, margarine and lemon juice. Tie cinnamon sticks and cloves in cheesecloth and add to syrup mixture. Simmer 15 minutes, stirring occasionally. Remove cheesecloth bag. Pour syrup over peaches. Bake, uncovered at 350° for 45 minutes. Serve warm with syrup. Makes 4 servings (1-1/2 peach halves per serving.)

Each serving equals: 1 FRUIT
                             1 SALTED FAT
                             1 CALORIE BOOSTER

CHERRY POT PIE

1 Cup Sugar
1 Cup Flour
3/4 Cup Milk
1-1/2 Teaspoon Baking Powder
1/2 Cup Margarine
1/2 Cup Sugar
One 16-Ounce Can Sour or Dark Sweet Cherries, Undrained
1/4 Teaspoon Almond Extract
Few Drops Red Food Coloring

Combine 1 cup sugar, flour, milk and baking powder. Melt margarine in a 1-1/2-quart casserole. Pour batter evenly over margarine. Mix 1/2 cup sugar, cherries, almond extract and food coloring. Pour on top of batter. Bake at 350° for 50 to 60 minutes. Makes 9 servings.

Each serving equals: 1 SALTED STARCH
                           1/2 FRUIT
                           2 CALORIE BOOSTERS

CRANBERRY NUT PUDDING

2-1/2 Cups Cranberries
  (Fresh or Frozen)
2/3 Cup Brown Sugar*
1/3 Cup Water
6 Tablespoons Margarine, Softened
1/3 Cup Sugar
1 Egg
1/2 Cup Flour
1/4 Teaspoon Allspice
1/3 Cup Chopped Walnuts*

Combine cranberries, brown sugar and water in a saucepan. Bring to a boil and cook, stirring until cranberries pop, about 5 minutes. Divide between eight 6-ounce custard cups, about 1/4 cup each. Beat margarine and sugar until fluffy. Beat in egg. Stir in flour and allspice, fold in walnuts. Spoon batter, about 2 tablespoons each, into berry-filled custard cups, dividing batter evenly. Place custard cups on a cookie sheet. Bake at 350° for 18 to 20 minutes. Serve warm. Makes 8 servings.

Each serving equals: **1 SALTED STARCH**
                                1/2 FRUIT
                                1 CALORIE BOOSTER

* Brown sugar and walnuts have been specially
  calculated into this recipe. Use them only as directed.

PEACH COBBLER

One 1 Pound 13-Ounce Can
  Sliced Peaches
1/2 Cup Sugar
2 Tablespoons Cornstarch
1/2 Teaspoon Cinnamon
1/8 Teaspoon Nutmeg

1 Cup Flour
1 Tablespoon Sugar
2 Teaspoons Baking Powder
2 Tablespoons Margarine
1/2 Cup Milk

Drain peaches, reserving 1 cup syrup. In a saucepan, combine 1/2 cup sugar, cornstarch, cinnamon and nutmeg. Blend in reserved peach syrup. Heat, stirring constantly, until mixture comes to a boil. Stir in peaches. Pour into an 8-inch square baking dish. Combine flour, 1 tablespoon sugar and baking powder. Cut in margarine. Add milk, stirring just enough to moisten. Drop by spoonfuls over peach mixture. Bake at 475° for 15 minutes. Serve warm. Makes 6 servings.

Each serving equals: 1 SALTED STARCH
                             1 FRUIT
                             1 CALORIE BOOSTER

CRANBERRY FREEZE

1 Apple, Peeled and Chopped
2 Cups Fresh Cranberries, Coarsely Chopped
1/2 Cup Sugar
1 Cup Marshmallow Creme
2 Cups "Cool Whip"

Combine apple, cranberries and sugar. Let sit in covered bowl 4 to 5 hours. Fold in marshmallow creme and "Cool Whip". Place in an 8-inch pan, cover and freeze. Cut into 6 servings.

Each serving equals: 1/2 FRUIT
2 CALORIE BOOSTERS

CRANBERRY SHERBET

One 16-Ounce Can Cranberry Sauce
2 Tablespoons Lemon Juice
2 Tablespoons Sugar

Combine cranberry sauce, lemon juice and sugar. Freeze until firm. Remove to a chilled bowl. Beat until light and fluffy. Refreeze. Makes six 1/2-cup servings.

Each serving equals: 1 CALORIE BOOSTER

HOLIDAY FREEZE

One 3-Ounce Package Lime Gelatin
One 20-Ounce Can Crushed Pineapple
1-1/2 Cups Miniature Marshmallows
1-1/2 Cups Crushed Buttermints
3-1/2 Cups "Cool Whip"
1/4 Cup Sifted Confectioners' Sugar

Mix gelatin with crushed pineapple. Mix in marshmallows and buttermints. Cover and let sit 4 to 5 hours. Fold in "Cool Whip". Spoon mixture into serving dish or 9 x 9-inch pan. Refrigerate. Dust with confectioners' sugar. Makes eight 3/4-cup servings. May also be frozen.

Each serving equals: **1/2 SALTED STARCH**
                                   1/2 FRUIT
                                   3 CALORIE BOOSTERS

QUICK 'N EASY
CHOCOLATE ICE CREAM

2 Cups "Cool Whip", Thawed
1/4 Cup "Hershey's" Chocolate Flavored Syrup, Chilled

Fold chilled chocolate syrup gently into thawed "Cool Whip". Refreeze in container or individual covered serving dishes. Makes four 1/2-cup servings.

Each serving equals: **1/2 FRUIT**
                             1 CALORIE BOOSTER

PEPPERMINT ICE CREAM

1 Cup "Coffee Rich"
1/2 Cup Crushed Peppermint Stick Candy
2 Cups Marshmallows
2 Cups "Cool Whip"

Heat "Coffee Rich", 1/4 cup crushed candy and marshmallows until candy and marshmallows are dissolved. Freeze in refrigerator tray until firm, about 2 hours. Beat in a chilled bowl until smooth. Fold in remaining candy and "Cool Whip"; return to freezer tray. Freeze until firm, about 3 to 4 hours. Makes three 1-cup servings.

Each serving equals: **1/2 SALTED STARCH**
                             4 CALORIE BOOSTERS

STRAWBERRY SHERBET

One 10-Ounce Package Frozen, Sweetened Strawberries
1 Tablespoon Lemon Juice
1 Cup Crushed Ice
3/4 Cup "Coffee Rich"
1/2 Cup Sugar
Few Drops Red Food Coloring

Thaw strawberries just until they break into chunks. Place strawberries, lemon juice, crushed ice, "Coffee Rich", sugar and food coloring in a blender. Blend until smooth and sugar is dissolved. Pour into a covered dish. Freeze until firm. Makes 6 servings, 1/2 cup each.

Each serving equals: **1/2 FRUIT**
                             1 CALORIE BOOSTER

CREAMY FROSTING

1/4 Cup Margarine
3-1/2 Cups Sifted Confectioners' Sugar
4 to 5 Tablespoons Milk or Cream
1 Teaspoon Vanilla

Cream margarine. Add 1 cup of the confectioners' sugar and cream well. Add the remaining sugar alternately with the milk or cream, using just enough milk to give a slight gloss and good spreading consistency. Add the vanilla and mix well.

**1/12 of the
recipe equals:**   **2 CALORIE BOOSTERS**

CREAMY CHOCOLATE FROSTING

Follow directions for creamy frosting adding 1-ounce unsweetened chocolate, melted, with the vanilla.

**1/12 of the
recipe equals:**   **2 CALORIE BOOSTERS**

COFFEE BUTTER FROSTING

1 Tablespoon Instant Coffee
3 Tablespoons Hot Milk
1/3 Cup Margarine
3-1/2 Cups Confectioners' Sugar
1 Teaspoon Vanilla or Rum or Brandy Flavoring

Dissolve instant coffee in hot milk. Combine margarine, confectioners' sugar, 2 tablespoons of hot milk mixture and vanilla. Beat mixture until smooth and fluffy. If frosting seems too thick, gradually beat in a little of the hot milk. Makes enough to fill and frost a 2-layer cake.

Each serving of
frosting equals: **1 CALORIE BOOSTER**

CREAM CHEESE FROSTING

One 8-Ounce Package Cream Cheese, Softened
1 Tablespoon Margarine
1 Teaspoon Vanilla
3-1/2 Cups Confectioners' Sugar

Beat cream cheese, margarine and vanilla until creamy. Add confectioners' sugar; beat until light and fluffy. Spread thickly over top of cake. Makes 2-1/2 Cups.

Each serving of
frosting equals: **1 CALORIE BOOSTER**

SEVEN-MINUTE FROSTING

2 Egg Whites
1-1/2 Cups Sugar
1 Tablespoon Light Corn Syrup
1/3 Cup Water
1 Teaspoon Vanilla

Combine egg whites, sugar, corn syrup and water. Beat 1 minute with electric mixer to mix well. Cook over rapidly boiling water (water should not touch bottom of double boiler). Beat constantly, about 7 minutes, or until stiff peaks form when beater is slowly raised. Remove from boiling water, add vanilla and continue beating until frosting is thick enough to spread, about 2 minutes. Makes enough to fill and frost a 2-layer cake.

Each serving equals: **1 CALORIE BOOSTER**

VARIATIONS:
  COFFEE SPICE: **Add 2 teaspoons instant coffee, 1 teaspoon cinnamon and 1/2 teaspoon nutmeg with vanilla.**

  PINK PEPPERMINT: **Omit vanilla. Add 1/2 teaspoon peppermint extract and a few drops red food coloring. Fold in 1/4 cup finely crushed peppermint candy.**

MAIN DISHES

MAIN DISHES

MAIN DISHES

MAIN DISHES

BEEF RAGOUT

2 Tablespoons Margarine
1 Pound Lean Beef, Cut in 3/4-Inch Cubes
1/2 Cup Finely Sliced Onions
1/8 Teaspoon Garlic Powder
1 Cup Fresh Mushrooms
  (Slice Stems and Caps Separately)
1 Crumbled Bay Leaf
1 Teaspoon Parsley
1 Teaspoon Rosemary or Oregano
2 Teaspoons Orange Marmalade
Dash of Cinnamon
1/4 Teaspoon Pepper
1/4 Green Pepper, Sliced
1/4 Cup Water

Melt margarine in large skillet. Add beef cubes; brown well on all sides over high heat. Lower heat, add onions, garlic and sliced stems of the mushrooms. Saute until onions are tender. Add bay leaf, parsley, rosemary, marmalade, cinnamon and pepper. Cover and simmer over low heat 1-1/2 hours, or until tender. Check occasionally and add a little water if meat appears dry. Ten minutes before ragout is done, add green pepper and sliced mushroom caps. Cover and complete cooking. Serve over buttered noodles. Makes 5 servings, approximately 1/3 cup each.

Each serving equals: **2 OUNCES MEAT**
                             1 VEGETABLE

BEEF STEAK WITH ONIONS

1 Pound Round Steak, 3/4 Inch Thick
1/4 Cup Flour
1/8 Teaspoon Onion Powder
Dash Garlic Powder
1/4 Teaspoon Pepper
3 Tablespoons Margarine
1/2 Cup Water
3 Cups Finely Sliced Onions
1/4 Teaspoon Paprika

Cut steak into 6 pieces, coat each piece with flour mixed with onion powder, garlic powder and pepper. Brown in hot margarine. Add water, cover and bake at 350° for 1 hour. Top meat with onion slices, sprinkle with paprika. Add a little more water if necessary. Cover and continue cooking until meat is tender, about 30 minutes. Makes 6 servings.

Each serving equals: **2 OUNCES MEAT**
                              1 VEGETABLE
                              1 SALTED FAT

BEEF STROGANOFF

2 Cups Fresh Sliced Mushrooms
3/4 Cup Sliced Onions
3 Tablespoons Margarine
1-1/2 Pounds Round Steak
1 Cup Water

1 Teaspoon Dry Mustard
1/8 Teaspoon Pepper
2 Tablespoons Flour
1/4 Cup Water
1 Cup Sour Cream

Saute mushrooms and onions in large skillet in margarine until soft; remove from skillet and set aside. Slice the meat into strips the size of a pencil, 3 to 4 inches long, and brown in skillet. Reduce heat to simmer. Return vegetables to skillet and add 1 cup water, dry mustard and pepper. Cover and simmer 45 minutes or until meat is tender, adding more water if necessary. Combine flour with 1/4 cup water, stir until smooth. Stir into meat mixture and cook until sauce thickens, about 2 minutes. Reduce heat to low. Just before serving, stir in sour cream. Serve over hot buttered noodles. Makes six 1/2-cup servings.

Each serving equals: 3 OUNCES MEAT
1 VEGETABLE
1 CALORIE BOOSTER

CRANBERRY POT ROAST

2 Tablespoons Flour
1/2 Teaspoon Onion Powder
1/4 Teaspoon Pepper
3 Pound Chuck Roast
2 Tablespoons Oil
4 Whole Cloves

2-Inch Stick Cinnamon
1/2 Cup Water
One 16-Ounce Can Whole
    Cranberry Sauce
1 Tablespoon Vinegar
2 Tablespoons Water

Combine flour, onion powder and pepper, rub into roast, using all flour mixture. In a dutch oven, slowly brown meat on both sides in hot oil. Add cloves, cinnamon and 1/2 cup water. Cover tightly and simmer about 2-1/2 hours or until tender, adding more water if necessary. Spoon off fat. Mix cranberry sauce, vinegar and 2 tablespoons water; add to meat. Cover and cook 10 to 15 minutes more. Remove cinnamon; spoon off fat. Pass pan juices with meat.

Each ounce of meat equals: **1 OUNCE MEAT**
THE SAUCE IS FREE

EGGPLANT AND GROUND BEEF CASSEROLE

3/4 Pound Fresh Eggplant
1/2 Cup Flour
1 Egg
1 Tablespoon Milk
1/4 Cup Dry Bread Crumbs
1/8 Teaspoon Garlic Powder
3 Tablespoons Oil
1/2 Pound Ground Beef

2 Tablespoons Tomato Paste
(Canned Without Salt)
6 Tablespoons Water
1/2 Cup Mozzarella Cheese,
Grated*
1 Teaspoon Parsley
1/4 Teaspoon Pepper

Peel eggplant and cut in 1/2-inch slices. Stack between paper towels and press out moisture. Coat with flour, dip in a mixture of beaten egg and milk. Coat again with bread crumbs. Heat oil and garlic powder, add eggplant a few slices at a time and brown on both sides. Add more oil if necessary. Drain eggplant on paper towels. Brown meat in same pan, drain off fat. Add tomato paste, water, cheese, parsley and pepper; stir to combine. Arrange eggplant slices and meat mixture in alternate layers in a small casserole, ending with meat sauce on top. Bake at 375° for 45 minutes. Makes 4 servings.

Each serving equals: **2 OUNCES MEAT**
2 VEGETABLES
1 SALTED FAT
1 CALORIE BOOSTER

*Mozzarella cheese does contain salt. It has been specially calculated into this recipe. Use it only as directed.

GOURMET HAMBURGERS

1/2 Cup Minced Onions
2 Tablespoons Margarine
1 Pound Ground Beef
1/8 Teaspoon Pepper
Dash Thyme
1 Tablespoon Margarine
1/2 Cup Red Wine
1 Teaspoon Margarine

Saute onions in 2 tablespoons margarine until onions are tender. Mix onions with ground beef, pepper and thyme. Divide into 5 patties and pan fry in 1 tablespoon margarine until done to taste. Remove hamburgers to hot platter and deglaze the pan with red wine. Scrape up all pan juices and brownings and cook until reduced by half. Remove from heat, add 1 teaspoon margarine. Stir briefly and pour over hamburgers. Serves 5.

Each hamburger equals: **2 OUNCES MEAT**
1/2 VEGETABLE
1 SALTED FAT
1 CALORIE BOOSTER

ITALIAN PIE

3/4 Pound Ground Beef
1/4 Cup Chopped Onion
1/8 Teaspoon Garlic Powder
1/2 Cup Small Curd Creamed Cottage Cheese*
1/4 Cup Grated Parmesan Cheese*
1 Teaspoon Oregano
1/2 Teaspoon Basil
One 6-Ounce Can Tomato Paste (Canned Without Salt)
3/4 Cup (3 Ounces) Shredded Mozzarella Cheese
1 Cup "Coffee Rich"
2/3 Cup Biscuit Mix (See Recipe Page D 12)
2 Eggs
1/4 Teaspoon Pepper

Saute ground beef with onion and garlic powder until browned, drain. Lightly grease pie pan. Layer cottage cheese and parmesan cheese in pie pan. Mix cooked beef, oregano, basil, tomato paste and 1/2 cup mozzarella cheese; spoon evenly over top. Beat "Coffee Rich", biscuit mix, eggs and pepper until smooth. Pour into pie plate. Bake at 400° for 30 to 35 minutes, until golden brown and knife inserted halfway between center and edge comes out clean. Sprinkle with remaining mozzarella cheese. Let stand 5 minutes before cutting. Cut into 6 servings.

Each serving equals: 2 OUNCES MEAT
                             1 SALTED STARCH
                             1 VEGETABLE
                             1 CALORIE BOOSTER

* Cottage, parmesan and mozzarella cheese do contain added salt.
  They have been specially calculated into this recipe. Use only
  as directed.

LASAGNA

2 Tablespoons Oil
1/2 Cup Finely Chopped Onion
1/8 Teaspoon Garlic Powder
1 Pound Ground Beef
1 Pound Canned Salt-Free Tomatoes
One 6-Ounce Can Tomato Paste (Canned Without Salt)
1/2 Cup Water
1/2 Teaspoon Pepper
1/4 Teaspoon Basil
1/2 Teaspoon Fennel
1 Teaspoon Parsley
2 Teaspoons Sugar
9 Lasagna Noodles (1/2 Pound)
2 Eggs
1 Pound Cottage Cheese*
2 Teaspoon Parsley
1/4 Pound Mozzarella Cheese, Cut in Thin Slices*
1/4 Cup Grated Parmesan Cheese*

In a large heavy pan, saute onion, garlic and ground beef in oil. Stir frequently, breaking up ground beef, until beef is well browned. Add tomatoes, tomato paste and water, mash tomatoes with a wooden spoon. Add pepper, basil, fennel, 1 teaspoon parsley and sugar. Bring to boil, reduce heat. Cover and simmer, stirring occasionally, until thick, about 1-1/2 hours. In an 8-quart kettle, bring 3 quarts of water to a boil, add lasagna noodles, 2 or 3 at a time. Return to boiling; boil uncovered stirring occasionally, 10 minutes, or just until tender. Drain in colander; rinse under cold water. Dry on paper towels. In a medium bowl, combine eggs, cottage cheese and 2 teaspoons parsley, mix. In

LASAGNA

the bottom of an 8 x 10-inch baking dish, spoon 1/3 sauce, top with 5 noodles, overlapping. Spread with 1/2 of cottage cheese mixture and 1/2 of mozzarella cheese, repeat using remaining 4 noodles, cottage cheese, mozzarella cheese and sauce. Sprinkle with parmesan cheese. Cover with foil, tucking around edge. Bake 25 minutes at 375°, remove foil and bake 20 minutes longer until bubbly. Cool 15 minutes before serving.

Cut into 12 servings, each serving equals:
    2 OUNCES MEAT
    1 SALTED STARCH
    1 VEGETABLE

Cut into 9 servings, each serving equals:
    3 OUNCES MEAT
    1 SALTED STARCH
    1 VEGETABLE

* Cottage cheese, mozzarella and parmesan cheese do contain added salt. They have been specially calculated into this recipe. Use them only as directed.

LONDON BROIL

1 Pound Flank Steak
1-1/2 Teaspoons Oil
1 Teaspoon Lemon Juice
Dash Pepper
Dash Garlic Powder
1 Teaspoon Parsley

Wipe steak dry with paper towels. Combine oil, lemon juice, pepper, garlic powder and parsley; use half to brush on top of steak. Broil, 4 inches from heat, 5 minutes. Turn and brush with rest of the oil mixture and broil 3 to 5 minutes longer. To serve, slice very thin on diagonal across grain. Makes six 2-ounce servings.

Each serving equals: **2 OUNCES MEAT**

MEAT LOAF

2 Eggs, Beaten
1/2 Cup Milk
1/2 Cup Soft Bread Crumbs
1/4 Cup Chopped Onions
2 Tablespoons Chopped
  Green Pepper

1/4 Teaspoon Thyme
1/4 Teaspoon Marjoram
1/4 Teaspoon Pepper
1-1/2 Pounds Ground Beef

Combine all ingredients except ground beef. Add ground beef, mix well. Shape mixture into a loaf, place in a loaf pan. Bake at 350° about 1-1/4 hours. Makes 8 servings.

Each serving equals: **2 OUNCES MEAT**

BERRY-GLAZED MEAT LOAVES

Meat Loaf (Previous Recipe)
1/2 of a 1-Pound Can Whole Cranberry Sauce
3 Tablespoons Sugar
2 Teaspoons Lemon Juice

Prepare meat loaf mixture according to previous recipe. Shape into 4 loaves. Place in oblong baking dish. Combine cranberry sauce, sugar and lemon juice, set aside. Bake loaves at 350° for 45 minutes. Spoon on sauce; bake 15 more minutes.

Remove loaves to warm platter. Skim fat from sauce. Pour some sauce over meat loaves and pass remaining sauce. Makes 8 servings, 1/2 loaf per serving.

Each serving equals: **2 OUNCES MEAT**
                                  1 CALORIE BOOSTER

OVEN DINNER

1 Piece Aluminum Foil, 12 x 15 Inches
1 Medium Potato
1 Small Carrot
1 Medium Slice Onion
3 Ounce Beef Pattie
  (If You Divide 1 Pound of Ground Beef into 5 Patties,
  Each Pattie Will Be Almost 3 Ounces)
Pepper
Parsley
1 Tablespoon Margarine

Early in the day, peel and slice potato and carrot into thin slices (1/8 inch). Soak in a large pan of water. An hour before dinner, place beef pattie in the center of foil, sprinkle with pepper, top with onion slice and drained slices of potato and carrot, sprinkle with more pepper and parsley flakes. Top with margarine. Close tightly. Bake on a cookie sheet for 1 hour at 375°. Serves 1.

Oven dinner equals: **2 OUNCES MEAT**
                                 2 VEGETABLES
                                 1 SALTED FAT

PIQUANT LIVER AND ONIONS

1 Cup Thinly Sliced Onions
2 Tablespoons Margarine
1/4 Cup Flour
1/8 Teaspoon Pepper
1 Pound Thinly Sliced Liver
2 Tablespoons Margarine
3 Tablespoons Vinegar
1 Teaspoon Parsley

Cook onions in margarine until tender; remove onions and set aside. Dredge liver in flour seasoned with pepper. Melt 2 tablespoons margarine in pan and cook liver until done; put on hot platter. Pour off fat, add onion and vinegar to skillet. Heat and pour over liver. Sprinkle with parsley and serve. Makes 6 servings.

Each serving equals: **2 OUNCES MEAT**
                               1 SALTED FAT

POT ROAST OF BEEF

1-1/2 Pounds Round Steak
3 Tablespoons Margarine
1/2 Cup Diced Onions
1/4 Cup Diced Celery
1/4 Cup Diced Carrots
2-1/2 Tablespoons Flour
1 Cup Water

4 Tablespoons Tomato Paste
  (Canned Without Salt)
1 Bay Leaf
1/8 Teaspoon Thyme
1 Tablespoon Cornstarch
1/4 Cup Water

Heat 1 tablespoon margarine in skillet. Brown steak and remove to baking dish. Add remaining 2 tablespoons margarine to skillet. Add onions, celery and carrots, saute until tender, stirring frequently. Stir flour into mixture and cook several minutes, stirring frequently. Slowly add 1 cup water, stir and cook several minutes. Add tomato paste, bay leaf and thyme. Mix well. Mix cornstarch and 1/4 cup water and slowly add to hot vegetable mixture. Stir and cook till smooth and thick. Pour vegetable mixture over meat, cover and cook at 350° 2 hours or until tender. Slice meat and divide meat and vegetables into 8 equal servings.

Each serving equals: **2 OUNCES MEAT**
                                  1 VEGETABLE

HOT ROAST BEEF SANDWICHES

Follow pot roast of beef recipe, when meat is cooked, slice into thin slices and serve over bread. Makes eight 1/2-cup servings of meat in gravy.

**Each 1/2 cup of meat
in gravy equals:**   **2 OUNCES MEAT**
                                  1 VEGETABLE

SAUERBRATEN

1-3/4 Pounds Chuck Roast
1-1/2 Cups Water
1/2 Cup Distilled Vinegar
1/2 Cup Sliced Onions
2 Tablespoons Sugar
4 Peppercorns

1 Whole Clove
1 Bay Leaf
1/2 Sliced Lemon
1/4 Cup Margarine
2 Tablespoons Flour

Place meat in large bowl. Add water, vinegar, sliced onion, sugar, peppercorns, whole clove, bay leaf and sliced lemon. Cover; marinate in refrigerator for at least 4 hours or several days. Turn meat several times.

Remove meat from marinade, drain thoroughly. Strain and reserve marinade. Melt 2 tablespoons margarine in skillet, brown meat. Add 1 cup marinade (reserve the rest). Cover and simmer 2-1/2 to 3 hours or until meat is tender. If necessary, add more marinade. Remove meat to warm platter. Pour off liquid from pan and set aside.

Melt 2 tablespoons margarine in saucepan, blend in flour, stirring constantly until mixture is golden brown. Remove from heat. Gradually add reserved cooking liquid, marinade and enough water to make 1-1/2 cups liquid. Return to heat, bring to a boil and cook, stirring constantly 1 to 2 minutes. Serve over meat. Makes 10 servings of meat and gravy.

Each serving equals: **2 OUNCES MEAT**

SHERRIED STROGANOFF

3 Tablespoons Margarine
1 Cup Sliced Onions
1-1/2 Cups Fresh, Sliced Mushrooms
6 Tablespoons Flour
1/4 Teaspoon Pepper
1 Pound Round Steak, Cut into Strips 1-1/2 Inches Long
1/2 Cup Sherry (Not Cooking Sherry)
1/4 Cup Water
3/4 Cup Sour Cream

Melt 1 tablespoon margarine in a large frying pan. Saute onions and mushrooms until tender. Remove vegetables and reserve. Add remaining margarine to frying pan. Toss beef strips in flour and pepper. Brown evenly in margarine, stirring often. Add sherry and water. Simmer covered for 45 minutes or until meat is tender. Mix in reserved vegetables. Slowly add sour cream, stir until smooth. Heat, but do not boil. Serve over noodles. Makes six 1/2-cup servings.

Each 1/2 cup serving equals: **2 OUNCES MEAT**
                                     1 VEGETABLE
                                     1 SALTED FAT

SPAGHETTI SAUCE

1/8 Teaspoon Garlic Powder
1/4 Cup Minced Onion
1 Tablespoon Margarine
1-1/2 Pounds Ground Beef
One 1-Pound Can Low-Sodium Tomatoes
One 6-Ounce Can Tomato Paste (Canned Without Salt)
1 Tablespoon Sugar
1 Teaspoon Basil
1 Teaspoon Oregano
1 Teaspoon Pepper
Water

Saute garlic and onion in margarine. Add ground beef and brown thoroughly. Using a wooden spoon, smash canned tomatoes. Add tomatoes, tomato paste, sugar, basil, oregano and pepper to ground beef. Simmer 30 minutes. Add enough water to make 4 cups sauce. Makes eight 1/2-cup servings.

Each serving equals: **2 OUNCES MEAT**
                                  2 VEGETABLES

STUFFED CABBAGE ROLLS

12 Cabbage Leaves
1 Pound Ground Beef
1/2 Cup Uncooked Long
   Grain Rice
1/4 Cup Grated Onion
2 Eggs, Beaten
1/4 Teaspoon Pepper
1/8 Teaspoon Allspice

2 Teaspoons Parsley
1/4 Cup Water
3 Ounces Tomato Paste
   (Canned Without Salt)
2 Tablespoons Lemon Juice
1 Cup Water
1/8 Teaspoon Pepper
1 Tablespoon Sugar

In large kettle, bring 3 quarts of water to a boil. Add cabbage, simmer 2 to 3 minutes, or until leaves are pliable. Remove cabbage and drain. Carefully remove 12 large leaves from cabbage, trim thick ribs. If inside leaves are not soft enough to roll, return to boiling water for a minute. In a large bowl, combine beef, rice, onion, eggs, pepper, allspice, parsley and 1/4 cup water. Mix together with a fork until well blended. Place about 1/4 cup meat mixture in hollow of each cabbage leaf. Fold sides of leaf over stuffing. Roll up from thick end of the leaf. Arrange rolls with seam side down in baking dish. Top with sauce made by combining tomato paste, lemon juice, 1 cup water and pepper. Bring cabbage rolls to boil over medium heat. Sprinkle with sugar; cover and bake at 375° for 1-1/2 hours. Uncover and bake 1-1/2 hours longer. Makes 6 servings, 2 cabbage rolls to a serving.

Each serving equals: **2 OUNCES MEAT**
                              2 VEGETABLES
                              1 CALORIE BOOSTER

STUFFED FLANK STEAK

1-1/2 Pounds Flank Steak
2 Tablespoons Margarine
1/2 Cup Chopped Celery
2 Tablespoons Minced Onion
2-1/2 Cups Bread Cubes
1 Teaspoon Parsley
1/4 Teaspoon Poultry Seasoning
1/4 Teaspoon Marjoram

1/8 Teaspoon Pepper
2 Tablespoons Margarine
2 Cups Fresh Sliced Mushrooms
1 Tablespoon Margarine
1/4 Cup Red Wine
1-1/2 Tablespoons Flour
1 Cup Water

Wipe steak with damp paper towels. Score in diamond pattern 1/8-inch deep on both sides. Melt 2 tablespoons margarine in dutch oven. Add celery and onion, saute until tender; remove from heat. Add bread cubes, parsley, poultry seasoning, marjoram and pepper; toss lightly. Place stuffing lengthwise down the center of the steak, roll and secure with skewers or tie. Melt 2 tablespoons margarine in dutch oven and saute mushrooms until tender, remove mushrooms from pan. Melt 1 tablespoon margarine in the dutch oven, add the steak and brown well on all sides. Spoon mushrooms and wine over steak, cover and bake at 350° 1-1/2 hours until tender. Remove steak to warm platter. Mix flour and water, add to mushrooms and meat juices. Heat to boiling, stirring constantly. To serve, cut steak crosswise, pour gravy over steak. Makes 8 servings.

Each serving equals: **2 OUNCES MEAT**
                              1 SALTED STARCH
                              1 VEGETABLE

STUFFED PEPPER CUPS

6 Medium Green Peppers
1 Pound Ground Beef
1/2 Cup Chopped Onions
1/4 Teaspoon Pepper
One 1-Pound Can Low-Sodium Tomatoes
1/2 Cup Water
1/2 Cup Uncooked Long Grain Rice
1/4 Cup Dry Bread Crumbs

Cut peppers in half lengthwise, remove seeds and membrane. Precook in boiling water 5 minutes, drain. Cook ground beef and onions until meat is browned. Add pepper, tomatoes, water and rice. Cover and simmer until rice is tender, about 15 minutes. Stuff peppers with meat mixture, place in baking dish. Top with bread crumbs. Bake, uncovered, at 350° for 25 minutes. Makes 6 servings, 2 halves per serving.

Each serving equals: **2 OUNCES MEAT**
                                  2 VEGETABLES
                                  1 CALORIE BOOSTER

CHICKEN BREASTS AND MUSHROOMS IN WINE

2 Tablespoons Margarine
2 Whole, Split, Chicken Breasts
2 Green Onions
1/8 Teaspoon Pepper
1-1/2 Cups Sliced Fresh Mushrooms
1/3 Cup White Wine or Vermouth (Do Not Use Cooking Wine)

Melt the margarine in a skillet and brown the skin side of the chicken. Turn chicken over, add the onions and saute for 10 minutes, until chicken is golden and onions tender. Season with pepper. Add mushrooms and wine, scraping any bits that are stuck on the bottom of the pan. Cover and cook over low heat for 20 minutes or until chicken is tender. Remove the chicken, onions and mushrooms to a warm platter. Cook the pan juices over high heat, stirring a few minutes to reduce. Pour over chicken and serve. Divide into 8 servings.

Each serving equals: **2 OUNCES MEAT**

CHICKEN CACCIATORE

2-1/2 Pounds Chicken Pieces
1/4 Cup Margarine
1/8 Teaspoon Garlic Powder
1/2 Teaspoon Italian Herbs

Cacciatore Sauce
(See Recipe Page I 4)

Brown chicken pieces in margarine and garlic powder. Sprinkle with Italian herbs, cover and simmer 40 to 50 minutes until tender. Prepare cacciatore sauce according to recipe. Serve hot sauce over chicken, accompanied by rice or noodles. Makes 5 servings.

Each serving equals:

2 OUNCES MEAT
1 VEGETABLE
1 SALTED FAT

CHICKEN CROQUETTES

1/4 Cup Margarine
1/4 Cup Finely Chopped Onion
1/3 Cup Flour
1 Cup Milk
1 Cup Chopped Celery

2 Cups Chopped Cooked
  Chicken
1-1/3 Cup Dry Bread Crumbs
1 Egg
2 Tablespoons Water

Melt margarine in small saucepan, add onion and saute until tender. Stir in flour and add milk. Cook over medium high heat, stir constantly until mixture thickens. Remove from heat, add celery and chicken. Spread mixture in shallow dish and chill 2 hours. Place bread crumbs on waxed paper. Beat egg with water in small bowl. Cut chilled mixture into 8 equal portions. Using spoon, drop and roll each portion in crumbs. Shape into cones. Coat with egg mixture and roll in crumbs again. Refrigerate at least 2 hours or overnight. Heat oil to 375° in deep fat fryer. Fry croquettes until golden brown, about 2-3 minutes. Drain on paper towels, serve hot with hollandaise sauce (See Recipe, Page I 7). Makes 8 servings.

Each croquette equals: 2 OUNCES MEAT
                            1 SALTED FAT
                            1 CALORIE BOOSTER

TURKEY CROQUETTES

Substitute 2 cups chopped, cooked turkey for chicken.

TUNA CROQUETTES

Substitute two 6-1/2-ounce cans of tuna, drained, for chicken.

CHICKEN PAPRIKASH

2-1/2 Pound Broiling Chicken, Cut Up
1/4 Teaspoon Pepper
1/8 Teaspoon Garlic Powder
2 Tablespoons Margarine
1 Cup Coarsley Chopped Onions
2 Medium Carrots, Thinly Sliced
1 Cup Water
1/2 Teaspoon Paprika
1 Cup Sour Cream
1 Teaspoon Parsley

Sprinkle chicken pieces with pepper and garlic powder. Brown a few pieces at a time in margarine in a large skillet. Remove chicken from skillet. Cook onions and carrots in same skillet for 5 minutes. Stir in water and paprika. Bring to a boil. Return chicken to pan. Cover and cook over low heat until chicken is tender, about 30 minutes. Transfer chicken to warm serving dish. Stir sour cream into sauce in skillet and heat, but do not boil. Pour sauce over chicken. Sprinkle with parsley. Makes 6 servings.

Each serving equals: **2 OUNCES MEAT**
                                                1/2 VEGETABLE

CHICKEN WITH WINE AND GRAPES

1 Tablespoon Flour
1/4 Teaspoon Pepper
2-1/2 Pound Chicken, Cut Up
6 Tablespoons Margarine
1/4 Cup Dry White Wine (Do Not Use Cooking Wine)
1/2 Cup Water
1 Teaspoon Parsley
1 Tablespoon Honey
1/4 Teaspoon Pepper
1 Bay Leaf
2 Tablespoons Grated Orange Rind
1 Cup Halved White Grapes

Combine flour and 1/4 teaspoon pepper, use to lightly dust chicken parts. Melt margarine in large skillet. Add chicken and saute over medium heat, until golden brown on all sides. Add wine, water, parsley, honey, 1/4 teaspoon pepper and bay leaf. Cover, simmer over low heat 15 minutes. Add orange rind. Continue cooking until tender (10-15 minutes). Remove chicken to serving platter. Add grapes to gravy and cook, stirring constantly, 2 minutes. Pour over chicken, Serves 5.

Each serving equals: **2 OUNCES MEAT**
                               1 SALTED FAT

LEMON BROILED CHICKEN

1/2 Broiling Chicken, Cut-Up
1/4 Cup Lemon Juice
2 Tablespoons Oil
1/4 Teaspoon Thyme
1/4 Teaspoon Marjoram
1 Teaspoon Grated Lemon Rind

Arrange chicken in broiler pan. Combine remaining ingredients, brush on chicken. Broil 6 inches from heat for 1/2 hour on each side, baste frequently with the lemon mixture. Makes approximately 5 ounces.

Each ounce of chicken equals:

1 OUNCE MEAT

THE BASTING SAUCE IS FREE

RICE-STUFFED CHICKEN

3/4 Cup Uncooked Rice
6 Tablespoons Margarine
1/2 Cup Chopped Onion
1/2 Cup Chopped Green Pepper
1/2 Teaspoon Sage
1/4 Teaspoon Thyme
1/8 Teaspoon Pepper
4 Pound Roasting Chicken
2 Tablespoons Margarine

Cook rice according to package directions, omitting salt. Melt 6 tablespoons margarine in skillet. Add onion and green pepper and saute. Combine cooked rice, sauteed onion and green pepper, sage, thyme and pepper. Toss lightly with a fork. Stuff chicken with rice mixture. Rub 2 tablespoons margarine on chicken. Bake at 325° for 2 hours. Baste occasionally with pan juices. Makes six 1/2-cup servings of rice stuffing.

Each serving of rice stuffing equals: **1 UNSALTED STARCH**
                                               1 SALTED FAT

Each ounce of chicken equals: **1 OUNCE MEAT**

SAUCY LEMON CHICKEN

1/3 Cup Lemon Juice
1/3 Cup Honey
1/4 Cup Minced Onion
1 Tablespoon Lemon Peel
1/2 Teaspoon Thyme
1/4 Teaspoon Pepper

2-1/2 Pounds Chicken Pieces
3 Tablespoons Margarine
1 Tablespoon Cornstarch
2 Tablespoons Water
1 Teaspoon Parsley

Combine lemon juice, honey, onion, lemon peel, thyme and pepper; pour over chicken and turn pieces to coat. Cover and refrigerate overnight or at least 4 hours, turning several times. Drain chicken and reserve marinade. Brown the chicken in a skillet in margarine. Place chicken and any remaining margarine in a baking dish. Pour reserved marinade over chicken. Bake, uncovered at 350° for 30 minutes, or until tender. Baste several times. When done, remove chicken to a serving dish. Blend cornstarch and water in small saucepan. Add remaining marinade from baking dish. Cook until thickened. Spoon off excess fat. Pour sauce over chicken and sprinkle with parsley. Makes 5 servings.

**Each serving of
rice stuffing equals:** **1 UNSALTED STARCH
1 SALTED FAT**

**Each ounce of
chicken equals:** **1 OUNCE MEAT**

SWEET AND PUNGENT CHICKEN

One 20-Ounce Can Pineapple Chunks
1/2 Cup Sugar
2 Tablespoons Cornstarch
1/2 Cup Vinegar
2 Tablespoons Diced Pimiento
2 Tablespoons Orange Marmalade
1/4 Cup Margarine
1 Pound Boned, Skinned, Chicken Breasts,
  Cut Into 1/2-Inch Cubes
1 Medium Green Pepper, Cut Into Thin Strips
1 Medium Onion, Thinly Sliced and Separated Into Rings

Drain pineapple, reserving 1/3 cup syrup. Combine sugar and cornstarch. Mix in pineapple, reserved syrup, vinegar, pimiento and orange marmalade. Set aside. Melt margarine in large heavy pan. Add chicken and cook for 5 minutes, stirring frequently. Add green pepper and onion; cook for 2 minutes. Add pineapple mixture. Bring to a full boil; stirring occasionally. Makes six 1/2-cup servings. Serve over rice.

Each serving equals: **2 OUNCES MEAT**
                              1 VEGETABLE
                              1 SALTED FAT

CHICKEN 'N ORANGE SALAD

1 Cup Chopped, Cooked Chicken
1/2 Cup Diced Celery
1/2 Cup Green Pepper, Chopped

1/4 Cup Finely Sliced Onion
1 Cup Mandarin Oranges
1/3 Cup Mayonnaise

Toss chicken, celery, green pepper and onion to mix. Add mandarin oranges and mayonnaise. Mix gently. Makes three 1-cup servings.

Each serving equals: 2 OUNCES MEAT
1/2 FRUIT
1 SALTED FAT

HAWAIIAN CHICKEN SALAD

1/2 Cup Diced Celery
1-1/4 Cups Shredded Head Lettuce
1-1/2 Cups Chopped,
  Cooked Chicken
1 Cup Drained Pineapple Chunks
1/2 Teaspoon Sugar

2 Teaspoons Lemon Juice
1/2 Cup Mayonnaise
Dash "Tabasco" Sauce
1/4 Teaspoon Pepper
Paprika

Place celery, lettuce, chicken and pineapple in a bowl. Mix sugar, lemon juice, mayonnaise, "tabasco" and pepper together; add to chicken mixture and toss to mix. Serve on a lettuce leaf. Sprinkle with paprika. Makes four 3/4-cup servings.

Each serving equals: 2 OUNCES MEAT
1 FRUIT
1 SALTED FAT

CHOPPED CHICKEN LIVERS

1 Pound Chicken Livers
2 Tablespoons Margarine
1/2 Cup Chopped Onions
1 Medium Carrot, Thinly Sliced
2 Tablespoons Sherry (Do Not Use Cooking Sherry)
2 Tablespoons Margarine
3 Hard Cooked Eggs
1/4 Teaspoon Pepper
Dash Paprika
Dash Ground Ginger
Dash Oregano
2 Tablespoons Mayonnaise

Wash livers and remove any discolored spots, drain. Heat 2 tablespoons margarine in fry pan, add onions and carrots and brown. When browned, add several drops of water and let sizzle. Scrape pan. Remove onions and carrots. Add the livers, sherry and 2 tablespoons margarine to the pan and cook for 10 minutes or until browned. Grind or chop onions, livers and eggs until smooth and pasty. Add pepper, paprika, ginger, oregano and mayonnaise. Mix until creamy. Makes seven 1/2-cup servings.

Each serving equals: **2 OUNCES MEAT**
                                 1 SALTED FAT

TURKEY BROCCOLI AU GRATIN

One 10-Ounce Package Broccoli
2 Cups Chopped, Cooked Turkey
1/3 Cup Margarine
1/3 Cup Flour
2 Cups "Coffee Rich"
1/4 Teaspoon Pepper
1/4 Cup White Wine (Do Not Use Cooking Wine)
1/4 Cup Grated Regular Cheddar Cheese*

Cook broccoli in boiling water until tender, drain. Lightly butter casserole dish. Layer 1/2 broccoli, 1/2 turkey, 1/2 broccoli and 1/2 turkey. Melt margarine in small saucepan. Remove from heat, stir in flour and pepper. Slowly add "Coffee Rich", stirring until smooth. Return to heat, stir until thick and smooth. Cook several minutes. Add wine, blend and remove from heat. Pour over turkey and broccoli. Top with cheese. Bake at 350° for 30 minutes, until bubbly. Makes 6 servings.

Each serving equals: **2 OUNCES MEAT**
                              1/2 VEGETABLE
                              1 SALTED FAT

* Regular cheddar cheese does contain salt. It has been specially calculated into this recipe. Use only as directed.

TURKEY GLORY SANDWICH

6 Ounces Cooked Turkey, Sliced Thin
6 Slices Bread
3 Tablespoons Margarine
8 Ounces Cream Cheese, at Room Temperature
1 Cup "Coffee Rich"
1/2 Cup Grated Parmesan Cheese*
1/8 Teaspoon Garlic Powder
1/4 Teaspoon Paprika

Toast bread and spread with margarine. Place turkey on toast. In a small saucepan, gradually mix "Coffee Rich" into cream cheese. Cook over medium heat till mixture begins to boil. Remove from heat and stir in parmesan cheese and garlic powder. Pour over sandwiches. Sprinkle with paprika and serve. Makes 6 sandwiches.

Each sandwich equals: **2 OUNCES MEAT**
                      1 SALTED STARCH
                      2 SALTED FATS

* Parmesan cheese does contain salt. It has been specially calculated into this recipe. Use it only as directed.

TURKEY NOODLE CASSEROLE

2 Tablespoons Margarine

1/4 Cup Chopped Onion

1/4 Cup Chopped Green Pepper

8 Ounces Cream Cheese

1-1/2 Cups "Coffee Rich"

1/4 Teaspoon Pepper

1/8 Teaspoon Garlic Powder

1/2 Cup Parmesan Cheese*

1 Cup Chopped, Cooked Turkey

2 Cup Cooked Noodles

1/4 Cup Dry Bread Crumbs

1/4 Teaspoon Paprika

Saute onion and green pepper in margarine till tender, remove vegetables from pan. Add cream cheese to pan and gradually mix in "Coffee Rich". Cook over medium heat just until boiling; remove from heat and add pepper, garlic powder and parmesan cheese. Stir in turkey and noodles, pour into 1-1/2-quart casserole dish. Sprinkle with bread crumbs and paprika. Bake at 350° for 15 minutes. Makes 6 servings.

Each serving equals: 2 OUNCES MEAT
1 UNSALTED STARCH
2 SALTED FATS

* Parmesan cheese does contain salt. It has been specially calculated into this recipe. Use only as directed.

CHICKEN NOODLE CASSEROLE

Follow recipe for turkey noodle casserole. Substitute 1 cup of chopped, cooked chicken in place of the turkey.

HUNGARIAN PORK CHOPS

1 Pound Trimmed Loin Pork Chops (Cut 3 to a Pound)
1 Tablespoon Oil
1/2 Cup Water
1 Teaspoon Paprika
1/2 Teaspoon Caraway Seed
1/2 Teaspoon Dill Weed
1/2 Teaspoon Onion Powder
1/8 Teaspoon Garlic Powder
2/3 Cup Sour Cream

Heat oil in frying pan, brown chops. Remove chops, drain off excess oil. Add 1/2 cup water, paprika, caraway seed, dill weed, onion powder and garlic powder to pan. Stir, scraping up browned bits from the bottom of the pan. Return pork chops to pan. Cover and cook on low heat for 1 hour or until chops are tender. Add more water if necessary. Remove pork chops to warm serving dish. Add sour cream to pan. Stir well and heat (do not boil). Serve sauce over chops. Makes 3 servings.

Each serving equals: **2 OUNCES MEAT**
                           1 CALORIE BOOSTER

PIZZA

DOUGH
- **1 Package Dry Yeast**
- **1/4 Cup Lukewarm Water**
- **1/2 Teaspoon Sugar**
- **2-1/4 Cup Flour**
- **1/2 Cup Lukewarm Water**
- **1 Tablespoon Oil**

In a small bowl dissolve yeast in 1/4 cup warm water with sugar. In a large bowl place 2 cups of flour; add yeast, 1/2 cup water and oil. Stir until mixture forms a soft dough. Knead dough on a surface floured with remaining 1/4 cup flour for 10 minutes until the dough is smooth and elastic. Transfer the dough to a large bowl, oiled lightly. Turn dough to coat with oil. Loosely cover with plastic wrap or a towel and let rise in a warm place for 1 hour or until double in bulk. Divide dough in half. Pat each half of the dough into a lightly greased pizza pan making a rim around the edge.

SAUCE
- **One 6-Ounce Can Tomato Paste (Canned Without Salt)**
- **1/2 Cup Water**
- **1/4 Teaspoon Garlic Powder**
- **1 Tablespoon Oregano**
- **1 Tablespoon Basil**
- **1/4 Teaspoon Pepper**
- **2 Tablespoons Olive Oil (Optional)**

Combine tomato paste, water, garlic powder, oregano, basil and pepper. Mix well. Spread half on each pizza crust. Sprinkle with olive oil, if desired.

PIZZA

TOPPINGS
  Italian Sausage (See Recipe Page F 39)
  1 Cup Sliced Fresh Mushrooms
  1/2 Cup Chopped Green Peppers
  1/2 Cup Chopped Onions
  8 Ounces Thinly Sliced or Grated Mozzarella Cheese*

Make sausage according to recipe using 1 pound ground pork. Cook, stirring, breaking up chunks until browned. Drain off fat. Spread evenly using half for each pizza. Divide mushrooms, green peppers and onions between pizzas and top with cheese. Bake at 425° for 15 minutes. Makes 2 pizzas. Cut each into 8 slices. Pizza may be frozen before cooking, cooked pizza is also good reheated.

Two slices equal: **2 OUNCES MEAT**
                            1 UNSALTED STARCH
                            1 VEGETABLE
                            1 SALTED FAT

Three slices equal: **3 OUNCES MEAT**
                            2 UNSALTED STARCHES
                            1-1/2 VEGETABLES
                            1 SALTED FAT
                            1 CALORIE BOOSTER

* Mozzarella cheese does contain added salt. It has been specially calculated into this recipe. Use only as directed.

ROAST PORK
WITH APPLES AND RAISINS

2-1/2 Pound Boneless Pork Roast (Tenderloin or Loin)
1/8 Teaspoon Pepper
1/8 Teaspoon Nutmeg
1/8 Teaspoon Allspice

SAUCE
  2/3 Cup Apple Juice
  1/2 Cup Raisins
  1-1/4 Teaspoons Cinnamon
  1/2 Cup Pork Drippings
  2 Cups Peeled, Cored and Diced Apples
  2 Teaspoons Cornstarch
  1/3 Cup Apple Juice

Rub roast with pepper, nutmeg and allspice. Place in baking pan and bake at 350° for 2-1/4 to 2-1/2 hours. Remove from oven and drain off pork drippings for sauce. Put roast back in oven to keep warm while preparing sauce.

Heat 2/3 cup apple juice in saucepan until warm. Add raisins, cinnamon, pork drippings and apples. Bring to a boil, stirring frequently. Mix cornstarch with 1/3 cup apple juice. Slowly add to the boiling apple and raisin mixture, stirring constantly while heating until thickened and smooth. Simmer for 5 minutes. Serve warm sauce over sliced meat. Makes 2-1/4 cups sauce and 24 ounces meat. Divide into 12 servings.

Each serving equals: **2 OUNCES MEAT**
                              1/2 FRUIT
                              1 CALORIE BOOSTER

SAUSAGE

1 Pound Lean Ground Pork
Desired Seasonings (See Recipes Below)

Mix seasonings thoroughly into ground pork. Refrigerate overnight. Make into 9 patties. Pan fry, bake or broil until done. Freeze uncooked patties individually until needed.

Each pattie equals: 1 OUNCE MEAT

ITALIAN SAUSAGE

1/4 Teaspoon Pepper
1/4 to 1/2 Teaspoon Crushed Red Pepper
3/4 Teaspoon Fennel

SPANISH SAUSAGE

1/8 to 1/4 Teaspoon
  Crushed Red Pepper
1/4 Teaspoon Garlic Powder
1/2 to 1 Tablespoon Chili Powder

1/8 Teaspoon Ground Cumin
1/2 to 1 Teaspoon Pepper
2 Tablespoons Vinegar

OLD-TIME COUNTRY SAUSAGE

1/2 Teaspoon Sage
1/8 Teaspoon Crushed Red Pepper
1/2 Teaspoon Pepper

NOTE: Use the lesser amounts of seasonings for milder sausage and the full amount for HOT sausage.

SWEET AND SOUR PORK

1 Pound Lean Pork, Cut Into 3/4-Inch Cubes
3 Tablespoons Margarine
1/8 Teaspoon Pepper
1 Cup Water
1/4 Cup Chopped Onions
4 Slices Canned Pineapple, Cut Into Segments
2 Medium Green Peppers, Cut in Strips
3 Tablespoons Cornstarch
1/4 Cup Sugar
1/4 Cup Vinegar
1/2 Cup Pineapple Syrup

Saute pork in margarine until well browned. Sprinkle with pepper, add water, cover and cook over low heat for 20 minutes. Add onions and pineapple, cook 10 more minutes. Add green peppers. Mix cornstarch and sugar, blend in vinegar and pineapple syrup. Add to pork mixture, stirring constantly until thickened. Simmer 5 more minutes. Makes four 2/3-cup portions. Serve over rice.

Each serving equals: 2 OUNCES MEAT
                             1 VEGETABLE
                             1 SALTED FAT
                             2 CALORIE BOOSTERS

BREADED VEAL CUTLETS

1/2 Teaspoon Paprika
1 Pound Thin Veal Cutlets (6 Pieces)
1 Cup Fine Dry Bread Crumbs, Unseasoned
1-1/2 Teaspoons Parsley
2 Eggs, Beaten
1/4 Cup Margarine
1/4 Cup Oil
Lemon Slices

Sprinkle cutlets with paprika. Pound cutlets with mallet to flatten. Combine bread crumbs with parsley. Dip cutlets into eggs then coat with bread crumbs. Place on wire rack to dry for 15 minutes. Fry in mixture of margarine and oil at 375° for 3 to 4 minutes on each side or until done. Drain on paper towels. Garnish with lemon slices. Makes 6 servings.

Each serving equals: 2 OUNCES MEAT
                              1 SALTED FAT
                              1 CALORIE BOOSTER

OSSO BUCCO

1/4 Cup Margarine
Dash Garlic Powder
2 Tablespoons Finely Minced Onion
1 Pound Sliced Veal Shanks
1-1/2 Tablespoons Flour
Dash Pepper
1/4 Cup Water
1/4 Cup White Wine
2 Tablespoons Tomato Paste (Canned Without Salt)
1-1/2 Teaspoons Parsley
1 Teaspoon Grated Lemon Rind

Melt margarine in heavy skillet, and garlic powder and onion. Saute onion until tender. Dredge veal shanks in flour and pepper, brown in margarine and onions on both sides. Add water, wine and tomato paste. Cover tightly and simmer slowly 1-1/2 hours until tender, adding more water if necessary. Sprinkle with parsley and lemon rind before serving. Makes approximately 4 serving, 2 ounces of meat each.

Each 2-ounce portion of meat and 1/4 of the sauce equals:

2 OUNCES MEAT
1 VEGETABLE
1 SALTED FAT

VEAL GOULASH

1/4 Cup Margarine
1 Pound Boneless Veal Cubes
3/4 Cup Chopped Onion
2 Teaspoons Paprika
2 Tablespoons Flour
1/4 Teaspoon Caraway Seeds
1 Bay Leaf
1/2 Teaspoon Parsley

1/8 Teaspoon Pepper
1-3/4 Cup Water
2 Tablespoons Tomato Paste
    (Canned Without Salt)
1 Tablespoon Cornstarch
1/4 Cup Water
1/2 Cup Sour Cream

Melt margarine in heavy skillet, add veal cubes and brown on all sides. Add onions and cook until transparent. Add paprika and flour. Stir and cook for 5 minutes. Add caraway seeds, bay leaf, parsley, pepper and 1-3/4 cup water. Bring to a boil. Cover and reduce heat, simmer slowly for 1 hour or until meat is tender. Mix tomato paste and cornstarch with 1/4 cup water. Add slowly, stirring constantly until sauce is thick and smooth. Slowly add sour cream, stirring constantly, do not allow to boil. Serve over noodles or rice. Makes six 1/2-cup portions.

Each serving equals: **2 OUNCES MEAT**
                             1 VEGETABLE
                             1 SALTED FAT

VEAL PICCATTA

2 Veal Shoulder Chops
1 Tablespoon Flour
2 Tablespoons Margarine
1 Tablespoon Lemon Juice
Dash Pepper
1/4 Teaspoon Parsley

Remove veal from bone, trim fat. Pound meat with a meat cleaver until the chops are as thin as possible. Coat chops with flour. Melt margarine and brown chops lightly on both sides. Sprinkle with lemon juice. Season with pepper and parsley. Serve with lemon wedges. Makes approximately three 2-ounce servings.

Two ounces equal: **2 OUNCES MEAT**

VEAL WITH SOUR CREAM

1/2 Cup Diced Onion
1/4 Cup Margarine
1 Pound Veal, Cut Into 1-Inch Cubes
1 Cup White Wine
1/8 Teaspoon Garlic Powder
2 Teaspoons Basil
1/4 Teaspoon Pepper
1-1/2 Cups Sour Cream

In a heavy skillet, saute onion in margarine until soft. Add veal cubes and brown on all sides. Add wine, garlic powder, basil and pepper. Simmer gently, covered, for 15 minutes or until the veal is tender. Add sour cream and cook slowly, stirring until sauce is blended and thickened, do not boil. Serve over rice. Makes six 1/2-cup servings.

Each serving equals: **2 OUNCES MEAT**
                       1 VEGETABLE
                       1 SALTED FAT

LAMB CURRY

1/4 Cup Margarine
2 Cups Chopped Onions
1/8 Teaspoon Garlic Powder
1 Pound Boneless Lamb Shoulder, Cut Into 2-Inch Cubes
One 8-Ounce Container Plain Yogurt
1 Teaspoon Ginger
2 Teaspoons Coriander
1/4 Teaspoon Cinnamon
1/2 Teaspoon Cardamon
1/4 Teaspoon Ground Cloves

Melt margarine in heavy pan, add onions and garlic powder. Saute until onions are tender and transparent, remove from pan. Add the lamb to pan and brown on all sides. Return the onions to the pan and add yogurt, ginger, coriander, cinnamon, cardamon and cloves. Simmer until tender, about 30 minutes. If desired, thin sauce with water before serving. Serve over rice. Makes five 1/3-cup servings.

Each serving equals: 2 OUNCES MEAT
                              1 VEGETABLE
                              1 SALTED FAT
                              1 CALORIE BOOSTER

SHISH KABOBS

1/4 Cup Minced Onion
2 Teaspoons Parsley
1/2 Teaspoon Marjoram
1/2 Teaspoon Thyme
1/4 Teaspoon Pepper
1/8 Teaspoon Garlic Powder
2 Tablespoons Lemon Juice
1 Pound Lean, Boneless Lamb,
　Cut Into 1-Inch Cubes

1 Green Pepper, Cut Into
　1-Inch Squares
1 Medium Tomato, Cut Into Chunks
2 Cups Small Whole Onions,
　Partially Cooked
1 Tablespoon Margarine, Melted

Combine onion, parsley, marjoram, thyme, pepper, garlic powder and lemon juice. Add meat, stir to coat. Refrigerate several hours or overnight, stirring occasionally. Alternate meat cubes and vegetables equally on 5 skewers. Place on broiler rack. Lightly brush vegetables with melted margarine. Spread on any remaining marinade mixture. Broil, about 4 inches from source of heat, turning once, until lamb and vegetables are tender and done, about 7 minutes per side. Makes 5 servings.

Each serving equals:　　**2 OUNCES MEAT**
　　　　　　　　　　　　　　　1-1/2 VEGETABLES

BAKED CRAB IMPERIAL

1/4 Cup Margarine
1/4 Cup Flour
2 Cups Milk
1/8 Teaspoon Pepper
1/2 Teaspoon Celery Flakes
Dash Cayenne
1 Egg Yolk, Beaten
2 Tablespoons Sherry
1 Cup Soft Bread Crumbs
1 Pound Flaked Crab
1 Teaspoon Parsley
1 Teaspoon Minced Onion
1/4 Cup Dry Bread Crumbs
1/2 Teaspoon Paprika

Melt margarine, remove from heat. Stir in flour. Gradually stir in milk; add pepper, celery flakes and cayenne. Stir and cook until thick. Add a small amount of white sauce to egg yolk and mix. Add egg yolk back to white sauce, cook 2 minutes. Remove from heat and gently stir in sherry, soft bread crumbs, crab, parsley and onion. Pour into casserole, top with bread crumbs and paprika. Bake at 400° for 20 to 25 minutes. Makes six 1/2-cup servings.

Each serving equals: 2 OUNCES MEAT
1 MILK
1 SALTED FAT

BROILED FISH

Arrange fish fillets in greased shallow baking pan. Brush lightly with melted margarine. Season with pepper, basil, garlic powder and a generous dusting of paprika. Broil 5 to 6 inches from heat until done through and golden. Allow 8 to 10 minutes for thin fillets and up to 15 minutes for thick. Serve with lemon wedges.

**Each ounce of
cooked fish equals:**   **1 OUNCE MEAT**

COQUILLES ST. JACQUES

1/2 Pound Raw Scallops
1 Tablespoon Margarine
2 Green Onions, Chopped
1/2 Teaspoon Parsley
1 Stalk Celery
1/8 Teaspoon Thyme
1 Bay Leaf
1/2 Cup White Wine
  (Not cooking wine)
1 Tablespoon Margarine

1/2 Cup Fresh Sliced Mushrooms
2 Tablespoons Water
1 Tablespoon Lemon Juice
1/8 Teaspoon Pepper
1-1/2 Tablespoon Flour
1-1/2 Tablespoon Margarine
1 Egg Yolk
1/3 Cup Heavy Cream
2 Tablespoons Parmesan Cheese
2 Tablespoons Bread Crumbs

Dry scallops on paper towels. Place in a saucepan with 1 tablespoon margarine, green onions, a boquet garni (a cheese-cloth bag) of parsley, celery, thyme and bay leaf. Barely cover with wine. Bring to a boil and simmer very gently for 4 or 5 minutes, or until scallops are just tender. Drain and save the broth, discard boquet garni. If large, cut the scallops in smaller pieces and set aside. Melt 1 tablespoon margarine in the saucepan, saute the mushrooms in it for a minute. Add water, lemon juice and pepper. Simmer mushrooms gently for a few minutes, then drain, combining the mushroom liquid with the reserved liquid from the scallops. Knead the flour with 1-1/2 tablespoons margarine, working them together into small balls the size of peas. Heat the reserved liquid from the scallops and mushrooms and gradually stir in the flour-margarine balls, one at a time. Cook and stir until the sauce is thickened and smooth, then cook for 2 to 3 minutes more. Add scallops and heat through. Beat the egg yolk with the cream, add the cream mixture to the sauce and cook gently, stirring until the sauce is very thick and smooth. Do not boil. Add the mushrooms. Spoon mixture into shells or individual dishes. Sprinkle with parmesan cheese and crumbs. Brown lightly under broiler and serve. Makes 3 servings.

Each serving equals: 2 OUNCES MEAT
                              2 VEGETABLES
                              2 SALTED FATS

CRAB RICE CASSEROLE

12 Ounces Salt-Free, Cooked Crab
3 Cups Hot Cooked Rice
1 Cup Shredded Cheddar Cheese*
One 3-Ounce Package Cream Cheese, at Room Temperature
1 Cup Sour Cream
1/2 Cup Chopped Onion
1/8 Teaspoon Garlic Powder
1/2 Teaspoon Basil
1 Medium Tomato, Sliced

Combine crab, rice and cheddar cheese. Spoon half of the mixture into a shallow 1-1/2-quart baking dish. Beat cream cheese until smooth. Stir in sour cream, onion, garlic powder and basil; spoon half over crab mixture. Layer with remaining crab mixture and top with sour cream mixture. Cover dish with foil, crimping the edges. Bake at 350° for 30 minutes. Uncover and top with tomato slices. Return to oven for 5 minutes. Makes 6 servings.

Each serving equals: 2 OUNCES MEAT
                             1 SALTED STARCH
                             1 SALTED FAT

* Cheddar cheese does contain salt. It has been specially calculated into this recipe. Use it only as directed.

FISH AU GRATIN

1 Pound Fresh or Frozen Unsalted Flounder, Sole or Haddock
1/3 Cup Mayonnaise
1/4 Cup Parmesan Cheese*
2 Tablespoons Dry Bread Crumbs

Brush each fish fillet with mayonnaise. Mix cheese and crumbs. Roll fish in crumb mixture, place in baking dish. Sprinkle with remaining crumb mixture. Bake at 375° until fish is lightly browned and flakes easily, 30 to 35 minutes for frozen fish or 25 minutes for thawed or fresh fish. Makes 5 servings.

Each serving equals: **2 OUNCES MEAT**
                             1 SALTED FAT

* Parmesan cheese does contain some salt. It has been specially calculated into this recipe. Use only as directed.

HaWaiian SHRiMP SaLaD

1 Cup Diced Celery
2 Cups Shredded Lettuce
1 Pound Raw Shrimp, Cooked
2 Cups Drained Pineapple Chunks
3/4 Cup Mayonnaise
2 Teaspoons Pineapple Juice
1/2 Teaspoon Sugar
Dash "Tabasco" Sauce

Combine celery, shredded lettuce, shrimp and pineapple chunks. Mix mayonnaise, pineapple juice, sugar and "Tabasco"; add to shrimp mixture and toss to mix. Makes five 3/4-cup servings.

Each serving equals: **2 OUNCES MEAT**
                              1 FRUIT
                              2 SALTED FATS

SALMON PATTIES

Two 7-3/4 Ounce Cans Low-Sodium Salmon, Drained
2 Eggs
2 Tablespoons Diced Onions
8 Squares Low-Sodium Crackers, Crushed
Dash Pepper
Dash "Tabasco" Sauce

Flake salmon. Add remaining ingredients. Form into 6 patties. Fry lightly on both sides in margarine or bake on a lightly greased cookie sheet at 350° for 15 minutes. Makes 6 patties.

Each pattie equals: **2 OUNCES MEAT**

SEAFOOD QUICHE

1-Crust Pie Shell (See Recipe Page E 1)
1/2 Cup Chopped Onion
1/4 Cup Chopped Green Pepper
1-1/2 Cups Sliced Fresh Mushrooms
2 Tablespoons Margarine
1/2 Cup Salt-Free Cooked Shrimp, Crab, or Tuna
1-1/2 Cups Shredded Swiss Cheese*
3 Eggs
1 Cup "Coffee Rich"
Dash "Tabasco" Sauce

Prepare pie crust as directed and place in 9-inch pie pan and set aside. Saute onion, green pepper and mushrooms in margarine until tender. Dice shrimp or flake crab or tuna and place in pie shell. Combine cheese, eggs, "Coffee Rich", "Tabasco" and sauteed vegetables; mix thoroughly and pour into pie shell. Bake at 350° for 50 to 60 minutes until brown on top. Serve immediately. Makes 6 servings.

Each serving equals: **2 OUNCES MEAT**
                             1 SALTED STARCH
                             2 SALTED FATS

* Swiss cheese does contain salt. It has been specially calculated into this recipe. Use only as directed.

SHRIMP AND FISH CREOLE

1 Cup Uncooked Long Grain Rice
One 7-Ounce Package Frozen Shrimp
1/2 Pound Frozen Cod
1-1/2 Cups Chopped Onion
1/2 Cup Chopped Green Pepper
1/4 Teaspoon Garlic Powder
1 Tablespoon Margarine
One 1-Pound Can Low-Sodium Tomatoes, Undrained
1 Tablespoon Parsley
2 Teaspoons Paprika
1/2 Teaspoon Sugar
1/8 Teaspoon Cayenne Pepper
1 Bay Leaf
1 Tablespoon Cornstarch
1 Tablespoon Water

Cook rice according to package directions, omitting salt. Partially thaw shrimp and fish. Saute onions, green pepper, and garlic in margarine until tender, about 5 minutes. Chop tomatoes and add with parsley, paprika, sugar, cayenne and bay leaf. Cover and simmer 30 minutes. Cut cod into 1-inch squares. Add to sauce with shrimp. Cook about 5 minutes, stirring occasionally, until the shrimp turns pink and the fish flakes easily with a fork. Mix cornstarch and water. Add to creole and cook, stirring constantly, until slightly thickened. Serve creole over cooked rice. Makes five scant 3/4-cup servings creole over 1/3 cup rice.

Each serving equals: **2 OUNCES MEAT**
                              2 VEGETABLES
                              1 UNSALTED STARCH

SHRIMP BROILED WITH GARLIC BUTTER

1 Pound Uncooked Shrimp
1/2 Cup Margarine
2 Teaspoons Lemon Juice
2 Tablespoons Minced Onions
1 Teaspoon Minced Garlic or 1/4 Teaspoon Garlic Powder
Dash Pepper
1 Tablespoon Parsley

Wash and dry shrimp. Melt margarine and add lemon juice, onions, garlic and pepper. Broil shrimp in garlic sauce 4 to 5 inches from heat for 5 minutes, turn and broil 5 more minutes. Serve on platter with strained pan juices. Sprinkle with parsley. Makes 5 servings.

Each serving equals: **2 OUNCES MEAT**
                                     1 SALTED FAT

TUNA NOODLE CASSEROLE

Follow the recipe for turkey noodle casserole, Page F 34, substituting one 6-1/2-ounce can of low-sodium tuna for 1 cup of turkey. Makes 6 servings.

Each serving equals: **2 OUNCES MEAT**
                                   1 UNSALTED STARCH
                                   2 SALTED FATS

TUNA RICE CASSEROLE

Substitute one 6-1/2-ounce can low-sodium canned tuna for crab in crab rice casserole recipe, Page F 52. Makes 6 servings.

Each serving equals: **2 OUNCES MEAT**
                                   1 SALTED STARCH
                                   1 CALORIE BOOSTER

TUNA PATTIES

Two 6-1/2-Ounce Cans Low-Sodium Tuna, Drained
2 Eggs
2 Tablespoons Diced Onions
8 Squares Low-Sodium Crackers, Crushed
Dash Pepper
Dash "Tabasco" Sauce

Flake tuna, add remaining ingredients. Form into 8 patties. Fry lightly on both sides in margarine or bake on a lightly greased cookie sheet at 350° for 15 minutes. Makes 8 patties.

Each pattie equals: **2 OUNCES MEAT**

TUNA MACARONI SALAD

See recipe page H 5.

VEGETABLE FISH BAKE

1-1/2 Cups Sliced Onions
2 Tablespoons Margarine
1 Pound Fillet of Sole
1/4 Teaspoon Pepper
1/2 Cup Sliced Fresh Mushrooms
1 Green Pepper, Sliced
1/4 Cup White Wine (Not Cooking Wine)
1 Tablespoon Lemon Juice

Arrange onions on bottom of 9-inch square baking dish. Dot with margarine. Season both sides of fish with pepper. Place on top of onions. Top with mushrooms and green peppers. Combine wine and lemon juice, pour over vegetables. Bake at 350° until fish flakes easily, about 25 to 30 minutes. Makes six 2/3-cup servings.

Each serving equals: **2 OUNCES MEAT**
                            1 VEGETABLE

EGG SALAD

1 Hard Boiled Egg
2 Tablespoons Mayonnaise
2 Teaspoons Diced Low-Sodium Pickles
Dash Pepper

Dice egg; add mayonnaise, pickles and pepper, mix lightly. Serve on lettuce, in a sandwich, or in a grilled sandwich.

Each serving equals: **1 OUNCE MEAT**
                             1 SALTED FAT

MEAT SALADS

2 Ounces Low-Sodium Salmon, Tuna, Chicken or Turkey, Diced
2 Tablespoons Mayonnaise
2 Teaspoons Diced Low-Sodium Pickles, if desired
Dash Pepper

Combine meat with mayonnaise, pickles and pepper. Serve on lettuce leaf, in a sandwich or in a grilled sandwich.

Each serving equals: **2 OUNCES MEAT**
                             1 SALTED FAT

SCRAMBLED POTATOES AND EGGS

2 Tablespoons Margarine
1 Cup Cold, Left Over, Specially Prepared Potatoes*
Dash Pepper
6 Eggs
1/2 Cup Light Cream
1/8 Teaspoon Pepper

Melt margarine in small skillet. Brown potatoes lightly in margarine. Sprinkle with pepper. Beat eggs, cream and 1/8 teaspoon pepper together lightly. Pour over potatoes. Stir until eggs are done. Makes 3 servings.

Each serving equals: **2 OUNCES MEAT**
                             1 SALTED FAT
                             1 CALORIE BOOSTER

*To make specially prepared potatoes, peel and slice potatoes into 1/8-inch slices. Soak in a large amount of water (5 cups for every cup of potatoes) 2 hours or overnight. Drain and cook in large amount of water (5 cups for every cup of potatoes) until tender. Drain and serve as desired.

FETTUCCINI ALFREDO

One 6-Ounce Package Fettuccini or Egg Noodles
1/2 Cup Light Whipping Cream
2 Tablespoons Margarine, Softened
Dash Pepper
1/2 Cup Grated Parmesan Cheese*

Cook noodles as directed on package, omitting salt. Drain well. Transfer to serving dish. Beat whipping cream, margarine and pepper until thick and creamy. Do not overbeat. Add parmesan cheese; pour over hot noodles and toss until evenly covered. Serve immediately. Makes four 1-cup servings.

Each serving equals: **1 OUNCE MEAT**
                             2 UNSALTED STARCHES
                             1 SALTED FAT

* Parmesan cheese does contain salt. It has been specially calculated into this recipe. Use only as directed.

MACARONI AND CHEESE

2 Cup Uncooked Elbow Macaroni
1/4 Cup Margarine
1/4 Cup Flour
1/8 Teaspoon Pepper
2 Cups Milk
8 Ounces (2 Cups) Grated Cheddar Cheese*

Cook macaroni in unsalted water until macaroni is cooked but firm. Drain and set aside. Melt margarine in saucepan, remove from heat, stir in flour and pepper. Gradually stir in milk. Stir until smooth, return to heat and continue to cook and stir until slightly thickened. Add 3/4 of the grated cheese. Combine with macaroni. Place mixture in 2-quart casserole and sprinkle evenly with remaining cheese. Bake uncovered at 350° for 30 minutes. Makes six 3/4-cup servings.

Each serving equals: **2 OUNCES MEAT**
                             1 UNSALTED STARCH
                             2 SALTED FATS

* Regular cheese does contain salt. It has been specially calculated into this recipe. Use only as directed.

MEAT COATINGS

BASIC MIX
- **1 Cup Dry Unseasoned Breadcrumbs**
- **1/4 Teaspoon Pepper**
- **1/2 Teaspoon Garlic Powder**
- **1/2 Teaspoon Basil**
- **1/2 Teaspoon Dried Celery Leaves**
- **1/2 Teaspoon Paprika**

Blend in blender or food processor until fine. To use, dip meat in melted margarine and coat with crumbs, one piece at a time, place meat in a pan and bake until done.

BEEF OR VEAL CUTLETS

Add 1/2 teaspoon marjoram or oregano to basic mix. Coat meat with melted margarine, then coat with mix, bake at 300° for 1 hour. Mix recipe is sufficient for 6 to 8 cutlets.

CHICKEN

Add 1/2 teaspoon thyme and 1/2 teaspoon sage to basic mix. Dip chicken pieces in melted margarine and coat chicken pieces with mix. Bake at 350° for 50 minutes. Mix recipe is sufficient for 1 cut-up chicken. Makes a wonderful oven-fried chicken.

PORK CHOPS

Add 1/2 teaspoon dried tarragon or 1/4 teaspoon allspice to basic mix. Coat chops with melted margarine, then with mix. Bake at 350° for 45 minutes. Mix recipe is sufficient for 6 pork chops.

**1/6 of meat coating
recipes equals:**   **1 SALTED STARCH**

VEGETABLES

DILLED GREEN BEANS

One 10-Ounce Package Frozen Green Beans
1/2 Cup Thinly Sliced Onion
2 Tablespoons Margarine
2 Teaspoons Dried Dill Weed
1/8 Teaspoon Pepper
1 Teaspoon Lemon Peel

Cook green beans and onion in boiling water until beans are tender, about 20 minutes. Drain. Stir in margarine, dill, pepper and lemon peel. Makes 3 servings.

Each serving equals: **1 VEGETABLE**
                              1/2 SALTED FAT

GREEN BEANS AND MUSHROOMS

Make gourmet green beans (below) omitting parsley. Saute 1 cup fresh sliced mushrooms in 1 tablespoon margarine and add to hot seasoned green beans. Makes 4 servings.

Each serving equals: **1 VEGETABLE**
                              1/2 SALTED FAT

GOURMET GREEN BEANS

One 10-Ounce Package Frozen Green Beans
1-1/2 Tablespoons Margarine
1 Teaspoon Lemon Juice
1 Teaspoon Parsley
Dash Pepper

Cook green beans in large amount of boiling water for 15 minutes. Drain, add margarine, lemon juice, parsley and pepper. Toss green beans to coat well. Makes 3 servings.

Each serving equals: **1 VEGETABLE**
                              1/2 SALTED FAT

SAVORY BRUSSELS SPROUTS

2 Cups Brussels Sprouts
1/4 Cup Margarine
1/4 Teaspoon Pepper
1/2 Teaspoon Lemon Juice

Trim brussels sprouts. Cook in large amount of boiling water for 5 minutes; drain. Add margarine, cook and shake well for 3 to 4 minutes to coat well. Add pepper and lemon juice. Makes six 1/4-cup servings.

Each serving equals: 1 VEGETABLE
                             1/2 SALTED FAT

HARVARD BEETS

1 Pound Can Low-Sodium Beets   1/3 Cup Water
2 Tablespoons Sugar   1/4 Cup Vinegar
1 Tablespoon Cornstarch   2 Tablespoons Margarine

Drain beets. In saucepan, combine sugar and cornstarch. Stir in water, vinegar and margarine. Cook and stir until mixture thickens and bubbles. Add beets, heat through. Makes three 1/2-cup servings.

Each serving equals: 1 VEGETABLE
                             1 SALTED FAT

FRIED CABBAGE AND NOODLES

1-1/2 Cups Cabbage (About 1/8 Head Raw)
1/2 Cup Dry Noodles
2 Tablespoons Margarine
1/4 Teaspoon Onion Powder
1/4 to 1/2 Teaspoon Caraway Seeds

Separate the cabbage leaves, rinse to clean. Soak in large amount of warm water for 2 hours; drain. Boil in large amount of water for 15 minutes; drain. Cook noodles in unsalted boiling water until tender; drain. Dice the cabbage into fairly small pieces. Melt margarine in a large frying pan. Add cooked cabbage and onion powder. Fry, until cabbage begins to brown slightly (about 15 minutes). Add the noodles and caraway seeds. Heat thoroughly and serve. Makes four slightly heaping 1/2-cup servings.

Each serving equals: 1 SALTED STARCH

HOT CABBAGE SLAW

2 Tablespoons Sugar
1 Tablespoon Minced Onion
1/2 Teaspoon Caraway Seed
1/2 Teapoon Dry Mustard
1/4 Teaspoon Pepper

3 Tablespoons Vinegar
2 Tablespoons Margarine
4 Cups Finely Shredded Cabbage
1 Cup Unpeeled Diced Apple

Combine sugar, onion, caraway seed, dry mustard, pepper and vinegar. Blend thoroughly and set aside. In a large skillet melt margarine. Add cabbage and apple, saute over medium heat for 3 minutes. Stir in vinegar mixture and simmer on low heat stirring occasionally, until apples and cabbage are tender, (about 5 minutes.) Makes 6 servings.

Each serving equals: **1 VEGETABLE**

GLAZED CARROTS

2 Tablespoons Margarine
1/3 Cup Brown Sugar*
2 Cups Cooked, Sliced Carrots

Heat margarine and brown sugar until sugar dissolves. Add carrots. Cook over medium heat, turning carrots until well glazed and tender, about 12 minutes. Makes six 1/3-cup servings.

Each serving equals: **1 VEGETABLE**
                             1/2 SALTED FAT

* Brown sugar is high in potassium, it has been specially calculated into this recipe. Use only as directed.

HOT DEVILED CARROTS

2 Tablespoons Margarine
2 Cups Cooked Sliced Carrots
1-1/2 Tablespoons Brown Sugar*
1 Teaspoon Dry Mustard
Dash "Tabasco" Sauce
Dash Pepper

Melt margarine in saucepan; add carrots and cook 3 minutes over low heat, until coated with margarine. Add brown sugar, mustard, "Tabasco" and pepper; mix well. Cover and cook over low heat for 5 minutes, stirring frequently. Makes four 1/2-cup servings.

Each serving equals: **1 VEGETABLE**
1/2 SALTED FAT

* Brown sugar is high in potassium, it has been specially calculated into this recipe. Use only as directed.

LEMON CARROTS

3 Cups Cooked Sliced Carrots
1 Tablespoon Sugar
2 Tablespoons Margarine
1 Tablespoon Lemon Juice
1/4 Teaspoon Grated Lemon Peel

Cook carrots in large amount of water until just tender, drain well. Add sugar, margarine, lemon juice and lemon peel. Heat and stir until margarine is melted. Makes six 1/2-cup servings.

Each serving equals: 1 VEGETABLE

CARROTS VICHY

2 Cups Sliced Carrots   1/8 Teaspoon Marjoram
2 Tablespoons Margarine   1 Teaspoon Parsley
1/4 Teaspoon Sugar

Cook carrots until just tender in large amount of water, drain. Add margarine and shake to coat well. Add sugar and marjoram, sprinkle with parsley. Makes four 1/2-cup servings.

Each serving equals: 1 VEGETABLE
**   1/2 SALTED FAT**

CURRIED CORN

One 10-Ounce Package Frozen Corn
2 Tablespoons Margarine
3/4 Teaspoon Curry Powder

Cook corn and drain. Add margarine and curry powder. Stir until margarine is melted and curry powder is thoroughly mixed. Makes four scant 1/2-cup servings.

Each serving equals: **1 VEGETABLE**
                              1 SALTED FAT

CORN PUDDING

2 Tablespoons Margarine
2 Tablespoons Flour
2 Cups "Coffee Rich"
One 16-Ounce Can Low-Sodium Whole Kernal Corn, Drained
2 Well-Beaten Eggs
1/2 Teaspoon Pepper

Melt margarine in a 1-1/2-quart casserole. Stir in flour to make a smooth paste. Add "Coffee Rich" very slowly, stir until smooth. Add corn, eggs and pepper. Set casserole in a pan filled with hot water 1 inch deep. Bake at 350° for 45-50 minutes until firm. Makes 4 servings.

Each serving equals: **1/2 OUNCE MEAT**
                              1 VEGETABLE
                              1 SALTED FAT
                              2 CALORIE BOOSTERS

FRIED POTATOES

4 Cups Specially Prepared Potatoes
1/3 Cup Margarine
1/2 Cup Chopped Onions
1/2 Cup Chopped Green Pepper
1/2 Teaspoon Pepper
1/4 Teaspoon Paprika
1 Tablespoon Parsley

Peel and slice potatoes in thin slices (1/8-inch thick) and soak in 5 quarts of water at least 2 hours or overnight. Drain well. Cook in 5 quarts of boiling water until just tender, drain well. Melt margarine in a large skillet. Add potatoes, onion and green pepper. Sprinkle with pepper and paprika. Cook, uncovered, over medium heat, about 20 minutes. Sprinkle with parsley just before serving. Makes six 1/2-cup servings.

Each serving equals: **1 VEGETABLE**
                              1 SALTED FAT

OVEN FRIED POTATOES

FOR EACH SERVING:
  1 Medium Potato
  1 Tablespoon Oil

OPTIONAL SEASONING:
  Dust with Paprika
  Pinch of Cayenne
  Pinch of Garlic Powder
  Pinch of Onion Powder

Peel potatoes and cut into french-fry strips. Soak at least 2 hours in a large pan of water (at least 5 cups water for 1 cup of potatoes). Drain and pat dry with paper towels. Measure 1 tablespoon oil into a bowl for each potato. Add potatoes and toss with a spoon, coating them lightly but thoroughly with oil. Spread the potatoes on a cookie sheet, not touching, and bake at 425° for 10 minutes, or until brown. Reduce heat to 350° and bake another 20 to 30 minutes, turning occasionally, until done through. Serve immediately, dust with seasonings if desired. Each potato makes one serving.

Each serving equals: 1 VEGETABLE
**   1 CALORIE BOOSTER**

POTATO CAKES

5 Cups Cooked Specially Prepared Potatoes
3 Tablespoons Minced Onion
3 Tablespoons Margarine
2 Tablespoons Milk
2 Eggs
1 Tablespoon Parsley
1/2 Teaspoon Celery Seed
1/4 Cup Flour
1/4 Cup Oil
1/4 Cup Margarine

Peel and slice potatoes into 1/8-inch slices. Soak in 6 quarts of water 2 hours or overnight. Drain and cook in 6 quarts of water until tender. Drain well. Saute onion in 3 tablespoons of margarine, add to potatoes and mash together with milk. Chill. Mix in eggs, parsley and celery seed. Divide mixture into 12 equal portions, shape into patties. Coat lightly with flour. Fry at 400° in oil and 1/4 cup margarine until browned on both sides. Makes 4 servings, 3 potato cakes per serving.

Each serving equals: 1/2 OUNCE MEAT
1 UNSALTED STARCH
1 VEGETABLE
2 SALTED FATS
1 CALORIE BOOSTER

POTATO PANCAKES

4 Large Potatoes, Pared
1/4 Cup Grated Onion
2 Eggs, Slightly Beaten
2 Tablespoons Flour
Dash Nutmeg
Dash Pepper
Oil for Frying

On a medium grater, grate potatoes. Drain well. Measure 3 cups of potatoes. Soak grated potatoes in 4 quarts of water at least 2 hours. Drain very well, pat dry with paper towels.

In a large bowl, combine potatoes, onion, eggs, flour, nutmeg and pepper. In a large, heavy skillet, slowly heat oil, 1/8-inch deep, until very hot but not smoking. For each pancake, drop 2 tablespoons potato mixture into hot fat. With spatula, flatten against bottom of skillet to make a pancake 4 inches in diameter. Fry 2 or 3 minutes on each side or until golden brown. Drain well on paper towels. Serve hot with applesauce or sour cream. Makes 12 pancakes.

Four pancakes equal: **1 MEAT**
                                    1 UNSALTED STARCH
                                    1 VEGETABLE
                                    1 CALORIE BOOSTER

SCALLOPED POTATOES

1-1/2 Pounds Potatoes
2 Medium Onions
2 Tablespoons Margarine
2 Tablespoons Flour
1/4 Teaspoon Pepper
1/8 Teaspoon Paprika
1-1/2 Cups "Coffee Rich"
1 Tablespoon Parsley

Wash, pare and thinly slice potatoes (about 4 cups). Soak potatoes in water (5 times more water than potatoes) for at least 30 minutes. Drain. Cook potatoes and onions, covered in a large amount of water (5 times more water than potatoes) until slightly tender. Drain. Melt margarine in saucepan. Remove from heat. Stir in flour, pepper and paprika. Blend in "Coffee Rich". Cook over medium heat, stirring until thick and smooth.

Layer one third of the potatoes and onions in a lightly greased 2-quart casserole, sprinkle with half the parsley, top with one third of the sauce. Repeat. Add remaining potatoes and onions, top with remaining sauce. Bake at 400° uncovered for 35 minutes or until top is browned and potatoes are tender when pierced with a fork. Makes six 2/3-cup servings.

Each serving equals:　　　**1 VEGETABLE**
　　　　　　　　　　　　　1 SALTED FAT
　　　　　　　　　　　　　1 CALORIE BOOSTER

SPICED SQUASH

One 12-Ounce Package Frozen Winter Squash
1 Tablepoon Margarine
1 Tablespoon Brown Sugar*
1/4 Teaspoon Grated Orange Peel
1/8 Teaspoon Cinnamon
Dash Cloves
Dash Nutmeg

Heat squash in top of double boiler until hot. Add margarine, brown sugar, orange peel, cinnamon, cloves and nutmeg. Stir until well blended. Makes four 1/3-cup servings.

Each serving equals: 1 VEGETABLE

*Brown sugar is high in potassium. It has been specially calculated into this recipe. Use it only as directed.

MIXED VEGETABLE SAUTE

2 Tablespoons Margarine
2 Cups Sliced Zucchini
1/2 Cup Diced Green Pepper
1/8 Teaspoon Garlic Powder
1-1/2 Cup Sliced Fresh Mushrooms
1/8 Teaspoon Pepper

Heat margarine in skillet. Saute zucchini, green pepper and garlic powder in margarine until vegetables are almost tender, stirring occasionally. Add mushrooms and pepper; saute about 10 minutes longer, stirring occasionally until vegetables are tender. Makes six 1/4-cup servings.

Each serving equals: 1 VEGETABLE

ZUCCHINI ITALIAN STYLE

1 Tablespoon Oil
1 Tablespoon Chopped Onion
1/8 Teaspoon Garlic Powder
1/2 Teaspoon Rosemary
4 Cups Sliced Zucchini
2-4 Tablespoons Water
1 Teaspoon Lemon Juice

Cook onion, garlic and rosemary in oil until onion is tender. Add zucchini and 2 to 4 tablespoons water. Cook 10 minutes just until tender. Blend in lemon juice, toss lightly. Makes six 1/2-cup servings.

Each serving equals: 1 VEGETABLE

MEXICAN RICE

3 Tablespoons Margarine
1-1/4 Cups Long Grain Rice
1/2 Cup Chopped Onion
1/4 Cup Diced Green Pepper
1/8 Teaspoon Garlic Powder
2-1/2 Cups Hot Water

One 1-Pound Can
   Low-Sodium Tomatoes
2 Teaspoons Chili Powder
1/4 Teaspoon Basil
1/4 Teaspoon Oregano
1/8 Teaspoon Pepper

Melt margarine in a large saucepan. Add rice, onion, green pepper and garlic powder. Cook, stirring, over low heat until rice browns. Add hot water, tomatoes, chili powder, basil, oregano and pepper. Bring to a boil. Cover and cook over low heat until liquid is absorbed and rice is tender, about 35 minutes. Makes seven 3/4-cup servings.

Each serving equals: 1 UNSALTED STARCH
                             1 VEGETABLE

MUSHROOM PILAF

2 Cups Fresh Sliced Mushrooms
1/2 Cup Chopped Onion
1/4 Teaspoon Garlic Powder
1 Tablespoon Parsley
1/2 Teaspoon Basil

1/8 Teaspoon Pepper
2 Tablespoons Margarine
2/3 Cup Long Grain Rice
1-1/3 Cup Water

Saute mushrooms and onions with garlic powder, parsley, basil and pepper in margarine, about 5 minutes, stirring frequently. Stir in rice and water. Cover and reduce heat. Simmer until liquid is absorbed and rice is tender, about 25 minutes. Makes four 3/4-cup servings.

Each serving equals: 1 UNSALTED STARCH
                             1 VEGETABLE
                             1/2 SALTED FAT

SALADS

APPLE GRAPE SALAD

2 Cups Diced Tart Apples, Unpeeled
2 Teaspoons Lemon Juice
3/4 Cup Diced Celery
3/4 Cup Halved, Seeded Grapes
1/4 Cup Mayonnaise
1/2 Cup "Cool Whip"

Sprinkle diced apples with lemon juice. Combine with celery, grapes and mayonnaise. Fold in "Cool Whip" and chill. Makes six 1/2-cup servings.

Each serving equals: 1 FRUIT
                             1/2 SALTED FAT

MARINATED BEAN SALAD

One 9-Ounce Package Frozen Green Beans
One 9-Ounce Package Frozen Yellow Beans
1/4 Cup Chopped Onion
1/2 Cup Distilled Vinegar
1/2 Cup Oil
1/2 Teaspoon Pepper
1/4 Cup Chopped Green Pepper
1/3 Cup Sugar
1/4 Teaspoon Dry Mustard

Cook beans and drain. Combine onions, vinegar, oil, pepper, green pepper, sugar and dry mustard; pour over beans. Cover and allow to marinate in refrigerator overnight. Makes six 2/3-cup servings.

Each serving equals: 1 VEGETABLE
                             1 CALORIE BOOSTER

PICKLED BEETS

1/2 Cup Vinegar
1/4 Cup Water
1/4 Cup Sugar
3 Whole Cloves
5 Black Peppercorns
2 Tablespoons Thin Onion Slices
2 Cups Low-Sodium, Canned Beets, Drained

Combine vinegar, water, sugar, cloves, peppercorns and onion slices in a saucepan. Add beets and bring to a boil. Serve hot or cold. Makes four 1/2-cup servings.

Each serving equals: 1 VEGETABLE

PINEAPPLE COLESLAW

1 Cup Finely Sliced Cabbage
1/2 Cup Drained Crushed Pineapple
1/2 Cup Packed Miniature Marshmallows
1/2 Cup "Cool Whip"
1/4 Cup Mayonnaise

Combine cabbage, pineapple and marshmallows. Combine "Cool Whip" and mayonnaise. Fold into cabbage mixture. Makes four 1/3-cup servings.

Each serving equals: 1/2 FRUIT
                                  1 SALTED FAT

TANGY COLESLAW

6 Cups Shredded Cabbage
1 Medium Carrot, Shredded
1/2 Medium Green Pepper, Chopped
3 Tablespoons Sugar
1/4 Cup Vinegar
2 Tablespoons Light Corn Syrup
2 Tablespoons Oil
1/4 Teaspoon Celery Seed
Dash Garlic Powder
Dash Onion Powder

Mix together cabbage, carrot and green pepper. Mix together sugar, vinegar, corn syrup, oil, celery seed, garlic and onion powder. Pour over cabbage mixture and marinate overnight. Makes 8 servings.

Each serving equals: 1 VEGETABLE

CREAMY CUCUMBER SALAD

3 Cups Thinly Sliced Cucumbers
1 Cup Thinly Sliced Red Onions
1/2 Cup Mayonnaise
1 Tablespoon Parsley
1 Teaspoon Lemon Juice
1/2 Teaspoon Sugar

Add mayonnaise, parsley, lemon juice and sugar to cucumbers and onions. Toss well. Makes 6 servings.

Each serving equals: 1 VEGETABLE
1 SALTED FAT

SWEDISH CUCUMBERS

2 Cups Sliced Cucumbers
2 Tablespoons Vinegar
1/2 Cup Sour Cream
1 Teaspoon Dill Seed
1-2 Drops "Tabasco" Sauce
1 Tablespoon Vinegar
2 Tablespoons Chopped Chives
Dash Pepper

Sprinkle cucumbers with 2 tablespoons vinegar. Let stand 30 minutes. Drain thoroughly. Combine remaining ingredients, pour over cucumbers. Chill about 30 minutes. Makes four 1/2-cup servings.

Each serving equals: 1 VEGETABLE

MACARONI VEGETABLE SALAD

1 Cup Uncooked Elbow Macaroni
1/4 Cup Chopped Celery
2 Tablespoons Green Pepper
2 Tablespoons Shredded Carrot
2 Tablespoons Minced Onion
1/8 Teaspoon Pepper
2/3 Cup Mayonnaise
1/2 Teaspoon Sugar
1 Tablespoon Lemon Juice

Cook macaroni in unsalted boiling water according to package directions, drain. Mix macaroni, celery, green pepper, carrot, onions and pepper. Stir in mayonnaise, sugar and lemon juice; chill. Makes eight 1/3-cup servings.

Each serving equals: 1 UNSALTED STARCH
1 SALTED FAT

TUNA MACARONI SALAD

Add one 6-1/2-ounce can Low-Sodium tuna and one chopped hard boiled egg to macaroni vegetable salad (above). Makes four 3/4-cup servings.

Each serving equals: 2 OUNCES MEAT
1 UNSALTED STARCH
1 SALTED FAT
1 CALORIE BOOSTER

HOT 'N HEARTY POTATO SALAD

4 Cups Special Potatoes, Cooked
1 Cup Chopped Onion
1 Tablespoon Margarine
1-1/2 Cups Mayonnaise

1/3 Cup Vinegar
1 Tablespoon Sugar
1/4 Teaspoon Pepper
1 Teaspoon Parsley

To prepare special potatoes, peel potatoes and slice into thin slices; soak in large amount of water (5 quarts) for at least two hours or overnight, drain and cook in a large amount of water (5 quarts) until tender; drain.

In a large skillet over medium heat, cook onions in margarine 2 to 3 minutes. Stir in mayonnaise, vinegar, sugar and pepper. Add potatoes; continue cooking, stirring constantly, about 2 minutes or until heated through. DO NOT BOIL! Garnish with parsley. Makes six servings, 3/4-cup each.

Each serving equals: 1 VEGETABLE
                              2 SALTED FATS
                              2 CALORIE BOOSTERS

POTATO SALAD

2 Cups Special Potatoes
2 Tablespoons Minced Onion
1/4 Cup Diced Celery
1/4 Cup Diced Green Pepper
1/8 Teaspoon Regular Horseradish
1/8 Teaspoon Dry Mustard Powder
2 Teaspoons Vinegar
1/8 Teaspoon Pepper
Dash Garlic Powder
3/4 Cup Mayonnaise

To prepare special potatoes, peel potatoes and dice into small cubes. Soak in large amount of water (10 cups) for at least two hours or overnight. Drain and cook in a large amount of water (10 cups) until tender; drain and cool.

Mix potatoes, onion, celery and green pepper together lightly. Mix horseradish, mustard, vinegar, pepper, garlic powder and mayonnaise together. Pour over potato mixture, toss lightly to mix. Sprinkle with parsley or paprika. Makes 3 servings, 3/4-cup each.

Each serving equals: **1 VEGETABLE**
                             2 SALTED FATS
                             2 CALORIE BOOSTERS

WALDORF SALAD

2-1/2 Cups Diced Apples, Unpeeled
1 Cup Diced Celery
1/3 Cup "Cool Whip"
2/3 Cup Mayonnaise

Combine apples and celery, fold in "Cool Whip" and mayonnaise.
Makes six 1/2-cup servings.

Each serving equals: **1 FRUIT**
                              1 SALTED FAT

SALAD DRESSINGS, SAUCES, RELISHES AND SHAKERS

SALAD DRESSINGS, SAUCES, RELISHES AND SHAKERS

BLUE CHEESE DRESSING

3/4 Cup Oil
1/4 Cup Vinegar
Dash Garlic Powder
Dash Pepper
1/4 Cup Crumbled Blue Cheese

Mix oil, vinegar, garlic and pepper. Chill. Add blue cheese and toss with salad just before serving. Makes 1 cup dressing.

One tablespoon equals: 1 CALORIE BOOSTER

CELERY SEED DRESSING

1 Cup Oil
1/3 Cup Vinegar
1/2 Cup Confectioners' Sugar
1 Teaspoon Celery Seed
1 Teaspoon Dry Mustard
1 Teaspoon Instant Minced Onion

Place all ingredients in a jar and shake well. Refrigerate. Makes 1-1/3 cups.

Two tablespoons equal: 2 CALORIE BOOSTERS

CREAMY ITALIAN DRESSING

3/4 Cup Mayonnaise
1 Tablespoon Red Wine Vinegar
1 Tablespoon Lemon Juice
1 Tablespoon Oil

1 Tablespoon Water
1/2 Teaspoon Oregano
1 Teaspoon Sugar
1/8 Teaspoon Garlic Powder

Combine all ingredients. Chill. Makes 1 cup.

Three tablespoons equal: 1 SALTED FAT
1 CALORIE BOOSTER

CREAMY ROQUEFORT DRESSING

1/2 Cup Mayonnaise
1/2 Cup Sour Cream
3 Tablespoons Milk
2 Tablespoons Lemon Juice

1/4 Teaspoon Paprika
1/3 Cup Crumbled Roquefort
(or Blue) Cheese

Combine all ingredients. Makes 1-1/2 cups.

Two tablespoons equal: 1 SALTED FAT
(LIMIT TO 2 TABLESPOONS A DAY)

PARISIAN DRESSING

1 Cup Mayonnaise
1/4 Cup Oil
1/3 Cup Red Wine Vinegar
2 Tablespoons Sugar

1 Teaspoon Paprika
1/2 Teaspoon Dry Mustard
Dash Garlic

Beat oil into mayonnaise. Add remaining ingredients and stir.
Makes 1-1/2 cups.

One tablespoon equals: 1 SALTED FAT

SWEET 'N SPICY DRESSING

1/2 Cup Oil
3/4 Cup Tarragon Vinegar
1/2 Cup Corn Syrup
1/2 Teaspoon Curry Powder
1/4 Teaspoon Pepper
Dash Cayenne
1/2 Teaspoon Onion Powder
Dash Garlic Powder

Combine all ingredients. Beat until blended and thick. Chill. Shake well before serving. Makes 1-3/4 cups.

Two tablespoons equal: 1 CALORIE BOOSTER

SWEET RED DRESSING

1 Cup Oil
3/4 Cup Sugar
1/3 Cup Vinegar
1/3 Cup Regular Ketchup*
1 Teaspoon Mustard Seed
1 Teaspoon Celery Seed
2 Teaspoons Minced Onion

Combine all ingredients in blender. Blend well. Makes 2 cups.

Three tablespoons equal: 1 SALTED FAT
1 CALORIE BOOSTER

*Regular ketchup does contain salt. It has been specially calculated into this recipe. Use only as directed.

CACCIATORE SAUCE

1/2 Cup Thinly Sliced Onions
1/2 Cup Diced Fresh Mushrooms
1 Tablespoon Margarine
1/8 Teaspoon Garlic Powder
1 Cup Low-Sodium Canned Tomatoes, Chopped
2 Tablespoons Tomato Paste (Canned Without Salt)
1/8 Teaspoon Pepper
1/2 Teaspoon Oregano
1/4 Teaspoon Basil
1 Bay Leaf
1/4 Cup Red Wine
2 Teaspoons Cornstarch
1/2 Cup Water

Melt margarine in a large skillet. Saute onions and mushrooms with garlic powder in margarine until onions are transparent. Add the remaining ingredients, cover and simmer for 1 hour. Serve as a sauce over fish, veal or chicken (which has been baked or broiled with an herb flavored margarine) with noodles or rice on the side. Makes 2 cups.

One-third cup equals: 1 VEGETABLE

CUCUMBER SAUCE

1/2 Small Unpeeled Cucumber
1 Cup Sour Cream
1 Teaspoon Dill Weed
1 Teaspoon Instant Minced Onion
1/4 Teaspoon Pepper

Shred cucumber, add remaining ingredients and mix. Refrigerate. Serve with tuna, salmon or other fish. Makes 1 cup.

One-quarter cup equals: **1/2 VEGETABLE**
                                             1 CALORIE BOOSTER

HERBED MARGARINE

1/4 Cup Margarine
1 Teaspoon Marjoram
1/8 Teaspoon Basil
1/8 Teaspoon Parsley
1 Teaspoon Dill Weed
1/2 Teaspoon Onion Powder
1/8 Teaspoon Garlic Powder
1/4 Teaspoon Paprika

Cream margarine until soft. In another bowl crush all the herbs against the side of the bowl with a spoon. Sprinkle the crushed herbs into the margarine and mix. Spread on bread, serve over vegetables or melt and pour over popcorn. Makes 1/4 cup.

One tablespoon equals: 1 SALTED FAT

NOTE: Herbs can be adjusted to individual taste.

HOLLANDAISE SAUCE

3 Egg Yolks
2 Tablespoons Lemon Juice
Dash "Tabasco" Sauce
1/2 Cup Hot, Bubbling Margarine

Put egg yolks, lemon juice and "Tabasco" in blender or food processor. Cover. Blend egg yolk mixture about 5 seconds, then add hot margarine in a steady stream, while continuing to blend. Blend until thick, about 30 seconds. Serve immediately over asparagus, broccoli, poached eggs, croquettes or fish. Makes 3/4 cup.

1-1/2 tablespoons equal: **1 SALTED FAT**
(LIMIT TO 1 SERVING A DAY)

MOCK HOLLANDAISE SAUCE

2 Tablespoons Hot Water
1/2 Cup Mayonnaise
1 Tablespoon Lemon Juice
Yellow Food Coloring

Blend hot water into mayonnaise in top of double boiler until blended and heated through. (Use wire whisk to blend.) Add lemon juice and a drop of yellow food coloring. Makes 2/3 cup.

Three tablespoons equal: **1 SALTED FAT**
1 CALORIE BOOSTER

SOUR CREAM SAUCE

2 Tablespoons Margarine
2 Tablespoons Chopped Onions
1/2 Cup Sour Cream
Dash Pepper

Saute onion in margarine until tender. Stir in sour cream and heat through. Do not boil. Serve over or mix with hot cooked vegetables. Sprinkle with parsley, if desired. Makes 1/2 cup.

Two tablespoons equal: **1 SALTED FAT**
                                  (LIMIT TO 1 SERVING A DAY)

VINAIGRETTE SAUCE

1/4 Cup Lemon Juice   **2 Tablespoons Vinegar**
1/2 Teaspoon Pepper   **5 Tablespoons Oil**
1/8 Teaspoon Garlic Powder   **1 Tablespoon Sour Cream**
1/4 Teaspoon Dry Mustard

Combine all ingredients and shake well. Pour over hot cooked vegetables or use as a marinade for chilled vegetables. Makes 3/4 cup.

Two tablespoons equal: **1 CALORIE BOOSTER**

CRANBERRY KETCHUP

1 Pound Fresh Cranberries
2 Cups Water
1-1/2 Cups Cider Vinegar*
2-1/2 Cups Sugar

2-1/2 Cups Brown Sugar*
2 Teaspoons Cinnamon
3/4 Teaspoon Ground Cloves
3/4 Teaspoon Allspice

In a large saucepan combine cranberries, water and vinegar. Bring to a boil and simmer for 5 to 7 minutes, or until cranberries have popped and are soft. Force the mixture through a sieve, pressing the pulp through the sieve with the back of a spoon. Discard the skins. Stir the sugar and spices into the pureed cranberries. Pour cranberries into a saucepan. Bring to a boil over moderately high heat stirring constantly. Boil for 10 to 15 minutes, or until ketchup is slightly thickened and 220°. Pour the ketchup into sterilized mason-type jars and seal. Makes about 3 pints. Use like regular ketchup.

Two tablespoons equal: **1 CALORIE BOOSTER
(LIMIT TO 1 SERVING A DAY)**

* Cider vinegar and brown sugar are higher in potassium than distilled vinegar and white sugar. They have been specially calculated into this recipe. Use only as directed.

HOT MUSTARD

2/3 Cup Dry Mustard
1/4 Cup Sugar
1/4 Cup Oil
1/2 Cup Wine Vinegar
1/2 Cup Water

Combine all ingredients; blend well. Refrigerate. Makes 1-1/2 cups.

Each serving is FREE

ZIPPY MAYONNAISE

Mix equal parts of mayonnaise and hot mustard.

Two tablespoons of
Zippy Mayonnaise equal: 1 SALTED FAT

HOLIDAY RELISH

2 Cups Fresh Cranberries
1 Whole Orange, Seeded and Diced
1 Apple, Unpeeled, Cored and Diced
2 Cups Sugar

Put fruits through food grinder or place in blender (1/2 cup at a time) and chop until coarsely grated. Mix in sugar. Refrigerate. Serve with pork or poultry. Makes 3 cups.

Three tablespoons equal: 1 CALORIE BOOSTER

RELISH

2 Lemons, Peeled,
  Quartered and Seeded
1 Cup Chopped Onions
1/2 Medium Green Pepper
1 Tablespoon Parsley
2 Cups Sliced Celery

1/2 Cup Sugar
1/4 Teaspoon Dry Mustard
1/8 Teaspoon Allspice
1 Teaspoon Celery Seed

Put lemons, onions, green pepper, parsley and celery through a food chopper, using a coarse blade. Stir in sugar and spices. Cover and place in refrigerator overnight to blend flavors. Makes 2 cups.

Two tablespoons equal: 1/2 FRUIT

SOUTH OF THE BORDER RELISH

1 Cup Finely Diced Tomatoes
1/2 Cup Minced Onion
1/2 Cup Finely Chopped Hot Peppers
  (Or Sweet Red Peppers, If Desired)
2 Teaspoons Vinegar
1/8 Teaspoon Garlic Powder
1/8 Teaspoon Grated Lemon Peel
1 Teaspoon Lemon Juice
"Tabasco" Sauce to Taste

Combine ingredients. Cover and refrigerate 8 hours. Makes 2 cups.

One tablespoon is FREE   (LIMIT TO 1 TABLESPOON A DAY)

DILL PICKLES

4 Pounds Cucumbers (4-Inches Long)
3 Cups Distilled Vinegar
3 Cups Water
3/4 to 1 Cup Dill Seed
18-21 Whole Black Peppercorns

Wash and slice cucumbers. Heat vinegar and water to boiling. Pack cucumbers into pint jars. Add 2 tablespoons dill seed and 3 peppercorns to each jar. Fill to within 1/2-inch of the top with boiling vinegar liquid. Seal and process in boiling water bath 20 minutes. Makes 6 pints.

Two tablespoons are FREE

SWEET PICKLES

1 Cup Water
1 Cup Cider Vinegar
1 Cup Sugar
1 Teaspoon Mace
3 Large Cucumbers, Sliced

Bring water, vinegar, sugar and mace to a boil. Add cucumber slices and simmer 6 minutes. Pour into a quart jar, cover and refrigerate. Makes 1 quart.

Two tablespoons are FREE

BREAD AND BUTTER PICKLES

Follow directions for sweet pickles, adding the following ingredients to the vinegar mixture, and bring to a boil:

1 Small Onion, Sliced and Separated Into Rings
1/2 Teaspoon Garlic Powder
1 Teaspoon Mustard Seed
1/4 Teaspoon Tumeric
Dash Cinnamon

Two tablespoons are FREE

HERB SHAKER FOR MEATS

1/4 Cup Parsley
1 Tablespoon Basil
1 Tablespoon Oregano
1 Tablespoon Paprika
1 Teaspoon Celery Flakes

Sprinkle herbs into blender. Set on low. Blend until well powdered. Store in airtight container.

SALAD HERBS

1/4 Cup Parsley
1/4 Cup Tarragon
1 Tablespoon Oregano

1 Teaspoon Dried Dill Weed
1 Tablespoon Celery Flakes

Sprinkle into blender set on low. Blend until well powdered. Store in airtight container.

HERB BLEND

1 Teaspoon Basil
1 Teaspoon Marjoram
1 Teaspoon Thyme
1 Teaspoon Oregano
1 Teaspoon Parsley

1 Teaspoon Nutmeg
1 Teaspoon Pepper
1/2 Teaspoon Savory
1/2 Teaspoon Ground Cloves
1/2 Teaspoon Cayenne

Combine and store in airtight container.

EACH SERVING IS FREE

NUTRITIVE VALUES OF RECIPES

RECIPE	Servings	Calories	Protein gm	Fat gm	Carbohy-drate, gm	Sodium mg	Potassium mg
Almond Flavored Shortbread	14	3080	31.0	187	320	2246	328
	1	220	2.2	13	23	161	23
Angel Pie	8	2663	20.1	94	448	1516	1446
	1	333	2.5	12	56	190	181
Apple Cheese-Filled Rolls	18	2829	48.5	168	309	1790	754
	1	157	2.7	9	17	99	42
Apple Crumb Pie	10	3281	27.0	145	477	761	988
	1	328	2.7	15	48	76	99
Apple Dumplings	8	3460	23.6	155	506	1052	1143
	1	433	3.0	19	63	132	143
Apple Grape Salad	6	740	2.6	53	68	455	817
	1	123	0.4	9	11	76	136
Apple Muffins	16	2042	36.9	72	315	770	1178
	1	128	2.3	5	20	48	74
Apple Nut Cobbler	8	3128	27.9	148	380	817	1492
	1	391	3.5	19	48	102	187
Apple Oven Pancake	2	806	17.4	36	104	492	366
	1	403	8.7	18	52	246	183
Applesauce Loaf Cake	10	3343	33.6	49	710	1246	1984
	1	334	3.4	5	71	125	198
Applesauce Raisin Coffee Cake	12	3177	40.2	131	472	1643	1330
	1	264	3.4	11	39	140	111
Baked Apples	6	1678	2.4	41	348	434	1157
	1	280	0.4	7	58	72	193
Baked Crab Imperial	6	1754	117.6	94	99	2892	2149
	1	292	19.6	16	17	482	358
Baked Spiced Peaches	4	1095	2.2	36	194	433	649
	1	274	0.6	9	49	108	162
Baking Powder Biscuits	12	1715	35.1	76	220	968	523
	1	143	2.9	6	18	81	44

RECIPE	Servings	Calories	Protein gm	Fat gm	Carbohy- drate, gm	Sodium mg	Potassium mg
Banana Split Dessert	9	2220	15.9	115	290	1507	1136
	1	247	1.8	13	32	167	126
Beef Ragout	5	1177	94.6	79	19	620	1817
	1	235	18.9	16	4	124	363
Beef Steak with Onions	6	1461	100.8	92	57	778	2074
	1	244	16.8	15	10	130	346
Beef Stroganoff	6	2283	150.3	168	34	604	2970
	1	381	25.0	28	6	101	495
Beef Coating Recipe	6	404	13.0	5	76	746	238
	1	67	2.2	1	13	124	40
Berry-Glazed Meatloaf	8	2622	142.3	161	145	733	2480
	1	328	17.8	20	18	92	310

Berry Pie (see Blackberry Pie, Raspberry Pie or Blueberry Pie)

RECIPE	Servings	Calories	Protein gm	Fat gm	Carbohy- drate, gm	Sodium mg	Potassium mg
Biscuit Mix	3-3/4 cups	2108	43.2	71	318	2109	390
Blackberry Pie	10	3788	39.5	181	510	293	1306
	1	379	4.0	18	51	29	131
Blonde Fudge	24	2214	8.2	40	457	291	362
	1	92	0.3	2	19	12	15
Blueberry Cake Muffins	18	2987	48.0	112	455	1748	737
	1	166	2.7	6	25	97	41
Blueberry Kuchen	16	2541	37.8	82	412	1552	631
	1	159	2.4	5	26	97	39
Blueberry Pancakes	10 pancakes	1235	30.9	51	165	1188	690
	1 pancake	124	3.1	5	17	119	69
	5 pancakes	618	15.5	26	83	594	345
Blueberry Pie	10	3812	36.7	179	524	293	794
	1	381	3.7	18	52	29	79
Blue Cheese Dressing	16	1576	7.2	174	4	481	47
	1	99	0.5	11	-	30	3
Brandy Alexander Pie	8	2519	15.2	111	296	1023	409
	1	315	2.0	14	37	128	51
Bread and Butter Pickles	64	997	9.7	1	251	63	1808
	1	16	0.1	-	4	1	28

RECIPE	Servings	Calories	Protein gm	Fat gm	Carbohy-drate, gm	Sodium mg	Potassium mg
Breaded Veal Cutlets	6	2272	113.4	168	76	1423	1732
	1	379	18.9	28	13	237	288
Bread Pudding with Raisins	4	1683	19.6	59	265	704	921
	1	421	4.9	15	66	176	230
Bread Pudding without Raisins	4	1463	17.8	59	207	684	368
	1	366	4.5	15	52	171	92
Broiled Fish	1 oz.	66	7.1	4	-	75	159
Brownie Mix	16 cups	11427	89.7	432	2061	3517	3757
Brownie Pudding	8	2073	25.0	33	439	977	1381
	1	259	3.1	4	55	122	172
Brownies	12	2273	25.8	134	261	1318	682
	1	189	2.2	11	22	110	57
Brown Mountain Cake	24	5167	75.7	216	730	3758	1272
	1	215	3.2	9	30	157	53
Butterscotch Wafers	8	738	0.1	12	162	241	12
	1	92	-	2	20	30	2
Cacciatore Sauce	6	284	5.7	13	34	174	1124
	1	47	1.0	2	6	29	187
Candy Chippers	12	2867	25.6	132	413	1830	823
	1	239	2.1	11	34	153	69
Carrots Vichy	4	305	3.1	24	23	387	706
	1	76	0.8	6	6	97	177
Celery Seed Dressing	10	2169	-	218	64	6	78
	1	217	-	22	6	1	8
Cherry Penuche	18	2544	4.8	27	576	545	248
	1	141	0.3	2	32	30	14
Cherry Pot Pie	9	2828	25.1	102	464	1661	1018
	1	314	2.8	11	52	185	113
Cherry Raspberry Pie	10	3522	34.4	155	503	15	1110
	1	352	3.4	16	50	2	11
Chicken Breasts and Mushrooms in Wine	8	888	122.4	36	11	542	2164
	1	111	15.3	5	1	68	271

RECIPE	Servings	Calories	Protein gm	Fat gm	Carbohy- drate, gm	Sodium mg	Potassium mg
Chicken Cacciatore	6	1172	90.1	72	34	966	2111
	1	234	18.0	14	7	193	422
Chicken Coating Recipe	6	403	13.0	5	75	746	240
	1	67	2.2	1	13	124	40
Chicken Croquettes	8	2843	122.3	192	152	1910	1908
	1	355	15.3	24	19	239	239
Chicken Noodle Casserole	6	2656	100.5	176	164	1751	1107
	1	443	16.8	24	27	292	185
Chicken 'N Orange Salad	3	849	47.0	64	25	618	1012
	1	283	15.7	21	8	206	337
Chicken Paprikash	6	1269	95.4	79	38	695	1912
	1	212	15.9	13	6	116	319
Chicken with Wine and Grapes	5	1354	86.6	83	56	1082	1424
	1	271	17.3	17	11	216	285
Chocolate Chippers	12	2556	25.6	131	333	1804	820
	1	213	2.1	11	28	150	68
Chocolate Fudge	9	2998	8.4	78	603	162	273
	1	167	0.5	4	33	9	15
Chopped Chicken Livers	7	1545	111.7	102	32	1273	1412
	1	221	16.0	15	5	182	202
Christmas Slices	18	3373	38.5	193	374	2309	413
	1	184	2.1	11	20	126	23
Cinnamon Pinwheels	12	2850	36.3	135	372	1677	578
	1	238	3.0	11	31	140	48
Coffee Butter Icing	16	2195	2.1	63	421	776	183
	1	137	0.1	4	26	49	11
Coffee Cloud Pie	8	2363	14.3	101	348	1572	565
	1	295	1.8	13	44	197	71
Coffee Penuche	18	2354	4.5	27	527	347	258
	1	131	0.3	2	29	19	14
Coffee Spice Frosting	16	1301	7.4	-	318	143	174
	1	81	0.5	-	20	9	11
Corn Muffins	18	1828	40.3	72	251	1237	712
	1	102	2.2	4	14	69	40

RECIPE	Servings	Calories	Protein gm	Fat gm	Carbohy-drate, gm	Sodium mg	Potassium mg
Corn Pudding	4	1489	25.9	82	158	669	793
	1	372	6.5	21	40	167	198
Coquilles St. Jacques	3	908	49.5	59	43	1357	1575
	1	303	16.5	20	14	452	525
Crab Rice Casserole	6	2046	111.3	117	126	2361	1777
	1	341	18.6	20	21	394	296
Cranberry Freeze	6	1646	3.1	34	334	154	407
	1	274	0.5	6	56	26	68
Cranberry Ketchup	48	4310	2.0	3	1100	185	2680
	1	90	-	-	23	4	56
Cranberry Kuchen	16	2494	37.0	82	400	1552	575
	1	156	2.3	5	25	97	36
Cranberry Nut Pudding	8	2194	21.1	104	268	955	1036
	1	274	2.6	13	34	119	130
Cranberry Pot Roast	32 oz.	4469	257.0	295	185	896	4262
	1 oz.	140	8.0	9	6	28	133
Cranberry Sherbet	6	760	0.7	1	196	5	178
	1	127	0.1	-	33	1	30
Cranberry Upside-Down Cake	12	2979	31.4	119	456	1849	880
	1	248	2.6	10	38	154	73
Cream Cheese Candy	7	1589	6.8	32	330	216	74
	1	227	1.0	5	47	31	11
Cream Cheese Frosting	16	2699	18.3	98	455	712	191
	1	169	1.1	6	28	45	12
Creamy Chocolate Frosting	12	2377	5.5	63	463	597	355
	1	198	0.5	5	39	50	30
Creamy Cucumber Salad	6	941	7.5	88	36	705	986
	1	157	1.3	15	6	118	164
Creamy Frosting	12	2197	2.5	48	455	596	120
	1	183	0.2	4	38	50	10
Creamy Italian Dressing	5	1329	2.0	146	10	985	107
	1	266	0.4	29	2	185	20
Creamy Roquefort Dressing	12	1220	16.1	126	11	1368	272
	1	102	1.3	11	1	114	23

RECIPE	Servings	Calories	Protein gm	Fat gm	Carbohy-drate, gm	Sodium mg	Potassium mg
Cucumber Sauce	4	471	7.6	43	11	105	333
	1	118	1.9	11	3	26	83
Curried Corn	4	421	8.5	27	52	564	545
	1	105	2.1	7	13	141	136
Dill Pickles	96	596	34.6	2	140	1194	3912
	1	6	0.4	-	1	12	41
Dilled Green Beans	3	312	5.7	23	21	293	562
	1	104	1.9	8	7	98	187
Easy Layer Cake	16	2288	29.9	78	366	1661	626
	1	143	1.9	5	23	104	39
Egg Salad	1	291	6.9	28	3	230	85
Eggplant and Ground Beef Casserole	4	1737	79.1	115	100	822	1955
	1	434	19.8	29	25	206	489
Festive Cranberry Torte	8	2869	17.5	92	501	137	355
	1	359	2.2	12	63	17	44
Fettucini Alfredo	4	1456	46.3	84	129	896	450
	1	364	11.6	21	32	224	112
Fish Au Gratin	5	970	77.7	68	12	941	1738
	1	194	15.5	14	2	188	348

Flavored Coffees (see Vienna, Orange and Mocha Flavored Coffees)

RECIPE	Servings	Calories	Protein gm	Fat gm	Carbohy-drate, gm	Sodium mg	Potassium mg
French Toast	6	739	33.8	23	94	1066	567
	1	123	5.6	4	16	178	95
Fried Cabbage and Noodles	4	390	7.3	25	36	313	221
	1	98	1.8	6	9	79	55
Fried Potatoes	6	1007	14.7	62	104	782	898
	1	168	2.5	10	17	130	150
Frosted Pineapple Cookies	12	2617	30.3	102	406	1504	465
	1	218	2.5	9	34	125	39
Frozen Chocolate Chip Cheesecake	10	3845	61.5	283	294	2672	1901
	1	385	6.2	28	29	267	190
Frozen Mint Pie	6	2081	7.6	123	234	1107	228
	1	347	1.3	21	39	185	38

RECIPE	Servings	Calories	Protein gm	Fat gm	Carbohy-drate, gm	Sodium mg	Potassium mg
German Coffee Cake	12	2075	28.4	69	335	1430	678
	1	173	2.4	6	28	119	57
Ginger Penuche	18	2416	4.5	27	543	545	219
	1	134	0.3	2	30	30	12
Glazed Carrots	6	574	3.0	24	93	404	946
	1	96	0.5	4	16	67	158
Glorified Rice	8	1405	7.4	56	204	80	307
	1	176	0.9	7	26	10	38
Gourmet Green Beans	3	234	4.4	17	15	214	420
	1	78	1.5	6	5	71	140
Gourmet Hamburgers	5	1705	84.5	135	15	768	1609
	1	341	16.9	27	3	154	322
Graham Cracker Pie Crust	Whole Recipe	1048	9.2	56	133	1321	455
Grasshopper Pie	8	2519	15.2	111	296	1023	409
	1	315	2.0	14	37	128	51
Greenbeans and Mushrooms	4	355	6.3	29	18	364	702
	1	89	1.6	7	5	91	176
Gumdrop Jumbos	18	6331	54.0	207	1093	3544	951
	1	352	3.0	12	61	197	53
Hard Candy	36	4412	-	-	1115	343	43
	1	123	-	-	31	10	1
Harvard Beets	3	449	2.8	23	61	416	507
	1	150	0.9	8	20	139	169
Hawaiian Chicken Salad	4	1357	69.6	95	58	867	1498
	1	339	17.4	24	15	217	375
Hawaiian Quick Bread	20	2172	43.1	76	329	1929	654
	1	109	2.2	4	16	96	33
Hawaiian Shrimp Salad	5	2020	87.6	137	120	1788	2170
	1	404	17.5	27	24	357	434
Herb Blend	8-1/2 tsp.	33	0.9	1	4	3	190
	1/4 tsp.	1	-	-	-	-	6
Herb Shaker for Meats	7 tsp.	61	2.8	-	12	17	435
	1/2 tsp.	2	0.1	-	-	-	10

RECIPE	Servings	Calories	Protein gm	Fat gm	Carbohy- drate, gm	Sodium mg	Potassium mg
Herbed Margarine	4	419	0.9	46	2	564	86
	1	105	0.2	12	1	141	22
Holiday Cranberry Bread	20	2616	46.2	67	452	1479	1083
	1	131	2.3	3	23	74	54
Holiday Eggnog	6	808	14.2	45	82	372	258
	1	135	2.4	8	14	62	43
Holiday Freeze	8	2743	11.2	61	546	815	628
	1	342	1.4	8	68	102	79
Holiday Relish	16	1808	3.1	3	460	12	502
	1	113	0.2	0	29	1	31
Hollandaise Sauce	8	999	8.9	108	3	1146	119
	1	125	1.1	14	-	143	15
Honey Orange Snack Bars	10	938	3.4	46	136	564	108
	1	94	0.3	5	14	19	4
Honey Taffy	13	1570	0.6	-	385	13	121
	1	117	-	-	29	1	9
Hot Buttered Rum	8	1113	0.7	46	185	606	548
	1	139	0.1	6	23	76	69
Hot Cabbage Slaw	6	496	5.5	25	66	355	1020
	1	83	0.9	6	11	59	170
Hot Cocoa	1	311	0.9	17	38	96	87
Hot Cocoa Mix	38	1302	19.5	40	232	331	1569
	1	34	0.5	1	6	9	41
Hot Deviled Carrots	4	377	3.0	24	42	388	779
	1	94	0.8	6	11	97	195
Hot Muffins	16	1876	36.6	72	271	768	614
	1	117	2.3	5	17	48	38
Hot Mustard	1-1/2 cups	683	-	55	55	7	504
	2 tsp.	19	-	2	2	-	14
Hot Roast Beef Sandwich	8	1827	143.3	120	29	988	3091
	1	228	17.9	15	4	124	386
Hot Spiced Cranberry Punch	5	811	0.9	-	211	9	211
	1	152	0.2	-	42	2	42

RECIPE	Servings	Calories	Protein gm	Fat gm	Carbohy- drate, gm	Sodium mg	Potassium mg
Hot Spiced Wine	3	317	0.2	-	40	6	466
	1	106	-	-	13	2	155
Hot 'N Hearty Potato Salad	6	3001	11.9	276	127	2142	911
	1	500	2.0	46	21	357	152
Hungarian Pancakes	10 pancakes	1174	17.9	52	152	319	314
	1 pancake	117	1.8	5	15	32	31
	5 pancakes	587	9.0	26	76	160	157
Hungarian Pork Chops	3	877	56.4	68	7	193	746
	1	292	18.8	23	2	64	249
Impossible Coconut Pie	8	3071	37.7	185	314	1652	1021
	1	384	4.7	23	39	207	178
Impossible Pumpkin Pie	8	1900	24.2	68	299	670	1277
	1	238	3.0	9	37	84	160
Italian Pie	6	2202	125.7	126	138	1549	2733
	1	367	21.0	21	23	258	456
Italian Sausage	9	1091	69.5	88	2	172	827
	1	121	7.7	10	-	19	92
Jam Bars	14	3097	32.7	102	513	1398	744
	1	219	2.3	7	37	100	53
Jelly-Filled Muffins	16	2132	36.6	72	335	769	619
	1	133	2.3	5	21	49	43
Jelly-Roll Cake	16	1788	32.7	23	368	565	531
	1	112	2.0	1	23	35	313
Knobby Apple Cake with Hot Lemon Nutmeg Sauce	12	3255	38.6	68	647	1677	1067
	1	271	3.2	6	54	140	89
Lamb Curry	5	1963	82.0	162	43	945	2061
	1	393	16.4	32	9	189	412
Lasagna	Whole Recipe	3672	240.0	186	260	2583	5081
	Cut into 12, 1 serving	306	20.0	16	22	215	423
	Cut into 9, 1 serving	408	26.7	21	29	287	565
Lemon Bavarian	6	1148	0.2	44	183	174	89
	1	191	-	7	31	29	15
Lemon Broiled Chicken	5 oz.	496	42.3	34	4	117	578
	1 oz.	99	8.5	7	1	23	116
Lemon Carrots	6	402	4.5	24	45	433	1057
	1	67	0.8	4	8	72	176

RECIPE	Servings	Calories	Protein gm	Fat gm	Carbohy- drate, gm	Sodium mg	Potassium mg
Lemon Drops	18	3479	42.9	108	594	1851	517
	1	193	2.4	6	28	103	29
Lemon Meringue Pie	10	3584	37.3	110	625	333	548
	1	358	3.7	11	63	33	55
Lemon Pudding	4	882	1.0	46	121	562	191
	1	221	0.3	12	30	140	48
Lemon Squares	24	4947	60.3	210	722	2641	791
	1	206	2.5	9	30	110	33
Lemon Tea Bread	20	3484	54.5	148	495	1734	903
	1	174	2.7	7	25	87	45
Light and Fruity Pie Strawberry	8	2233	18.4	114	278	1547	754
	1	279	2.3	14	35	193	94
Blueberry	8	2253	18.4	114	287	1547	627
	1	281	2.3	14	36	193	78
Raspberry	8	2218	18.9	114	282	1547	717
	1	277	2.4	14	35	193	90
Pineapple	8	2352	18.2	113	315	1549	755
	1	294	2.3	14	39	194	94
Lime Bavarian	6	1148	0.2	44	183	174	89
	1	191	-	7	31	29	15
Lime Snow	8	687	19.6	-	159	96	223
	1	86	2.5	-	20	12	28
London Broil	6	716	98.1	33	-	344	1589
	1	119	16.4	6	-	57	265
Macaroni and Cheese	6	2592	106.2	139	226	2399	1385
	1	432	17.7	23	38	400	231
Macaroni Vegetable Salad	8	1495	16.9	117	94	928	463
	1	187	2.1	15	12	116	58
Maple or Walnut Flavored Penuche	18	2352	4.5	27	527	545	206
	1	130	0.3	2	29	30	11
Marble Loaf Cake	24	3494	49.1	140	517	2455	1078
	1	146	2.0	6	22	102	45
Marinated Bean Salad	6	1390	9.0	109	104	15	938
	1	232	1.5	18	17	3	156

RECIPE		Servings	Calories	Protein gm	Fat gm	Carbohy- drate, gm	Sodium mg	Potassium mg
Meat Coatings (see Beef, Veal, Chicken or Pork Chop Meat Coatings)								
Meat Loaf		8	2151	142.0	161	23	730	2398
		1	269	17.8	20	3	91	300
Meat Salads	Salmon	1	286	12.0	26	2	205	225
	Tuna	1	278	16.3	22	2	192	178
	Chicken	1	300	18.3	24	2	205	253
	Turkey	1	314	18.3	25	2	243	228
Meltaways		18	4127	36.6	372	471	2252	677
		1	229	2.0	15	26	125	38
Mexican Rice		7	1291	22.6	37	208	461	1496
		1	184	3.2	5	30	66	214
Mint Bavarian		6	1006	0.1	44	146	173	38
		1	168	-	7	24	29	6
Mixed Vegetable Saute		6	304	6.9	24	17	310	1078
		1	51	1.2	4	3	52	180
Mocha Flavored Coffee		20	990	4.2	36	163	291	1593
		1	50	0.2	2	8	15	80
Mock Hollandaise Sauce		2/3 cup	793	1.3	88	3	657	59
		3 Tbsp	223	0.4	25	1	185	17
Moon Pies		18	3513	46.5	113	552	2740	1020
		1	195	2.6	6	31	152	57
Mushroom Pilaf		4	731	13.9	24	13	320	889
		1	183	3.5	6	28	80	222
Old-Fashioned Apple Pie		10	3841	32.3	178	531	296	1147
		1	384	3.2	18	53	30	115
Old-Fashioned Popcorn Balls		20	2184	3.8	2	544	116	164
		1	109	0.2	0	27	6	8
Old-Time Country Sausage		9	1093	69.4	88	1	172	798
		1	121	7.7	10	-	19	89
Onion Parsley Butterfingers		16	2085	34.7	140	179	2374	577
		1	130	2.2	9	11	148	36

RECIPE		Servings	Calories	Protein gm	Fat gm	Carbohy-drate, gm	Sodium mg	Potassium mg
Orange Flavored Coffee		20	1165	2.4	34	208	220	1540
		1	58	0.1	2	10	11	77
Orange Penuche		18	2476	4.6	27	558	545	226
		1	138	0.3	2	31	30	38
Osso Bucco		4	1127	71.7	77	24	778	1514
		1	282	17.9	19	6	195	378
Oven Dinner		1	450	19.0	30	28	225	565
Oven Fried Potatoes		1	208	2.6	14	20	3	200
Pancakes		10 pancakes	1144	29.7	50	142	1186	556
		5 pancakes	572	14.9	25	71	593	278
		1 pancake	114	3.0	5	14	119	56
Parisian Dressing		24	2152	2.7	231	30	1315	212
		1	90	0.1	10	1	55	9
Peach Cobbler		6	1941	22.2	29	404	943	1392
		1	324	3.7	5	67	157	232
Peanut Butter Fudge		10	2295	23.0	62	419	379	691
		1	230	2.3	6	42	38	69
Pear Peppermint Pie		8	2548	16.1	113	387	1400	900
		1	318	2.0	14	48	175	113
Penuche		18	2352	4.5	27	527	545	206
		1	131	0.3	2	29	30	11
Peppermint Ice Cream		3	1460	2.6	55	233	232	122
		1	487	0.9	18	78	77	41
Pickled Beets		4	348	3.4	-	88	160	635
		1	87	0.9	-	22	40	159
Pie Shell	2-Crust	Whole Recipe	2324	28.8	153	209	6	260
	1-Crust	Whole Recipe	1206	14.4	81	104	3	130
Pineapple Coleslaw		4	714	2.8	52	62	367	362
		1	179	0.7	13	16	92	91
Pineapple Upside-Down Cake		9	3362	22.0	139	514	2399	1041
		1	374	2.4	15	57	267	116

RECIPE	Servings	Calories	Protein gm	Fat gm	Carbohy-drate, gm	Sodium mg	Potassium mg
Pink Peppermint Frosting	16	1434	7.2	-	352	155	109
	1	90	0.5	-	22	10	7
Piquant Liver and Onions	6	1220	96.1	64	62	1191	1521
	1	203	16.0	11	10	199	254
Pizza	16 slices	3459	158.3	182	296	1111	3664
	3 slices	636	29.7	33	56	208	687
	2 slices	432	19.8	22	37	139	458
Popover Pancake	2	989	24.9	63	81	745	385
	1	495	12.5	32	41	373	193
Pot Roast of Beef	8	1827	143.3	120	29	988	3091
	1	228	17.9	15	4	124	386
Pork Chops Coating Recipe	6	407	13.1	5	76	746	259
	1	68	2.2	1	13	124	43
Potato Cakes	4	2026	33.7	150	145	1140	984
	1	506	8.4	38	36	285	246
Potato Pancakes	3	766	29.9	13	135	138	1020
	1	255	10.0	4	45	46	340
Potato Salad	3	1412	7.0	132	55	1037	498
	1	471	2.3	44	18	346	166
Puffed Rice Brittle	15	1374	2.7	-	339	3	54
	1	92	0.2	-	23	-	4
Pumpkin Bread	20	2533	49.0	66	435	1936	1202
	1	127	2.5	3	22	97	60
Pumpkin Pie	8	2805	26.2	122	402	268	1240
	1	351	3.3	15	50	34	155
Quick Biscuits	6	615	4.3	22	89	603	221
	1	103	2.4	4	15	101	37
Quick Cheesecake Dessert with Blueberry Glaze	8	2792	29.6	176	286	1913	882
	1	349	3.7	22	36	239	110
with Pineapple Glaze	8	2915	28.3	176	305	1912	885
	1	364	3.5	22	38	239	111

RECIPE	Servings	Calories	Protein gm	Fat gm	Carbohy-drate, gm	Sodium mg	Potassium mg
Quick Cheesecake Dessert with Red Cherry Glaze	8	2997	31.3	176	337	1919	1263
	1	375	3.9	22	42	240	158
with Strawberry Glaze	8	2946	29.0	176	326	1913	970
	1	368	3.6	22	41	239	121
Quick Cinnamon Bread	20	3287	43.6	92	570	1929	637
	1	164	2.2	5	29	96	32
Quick 'N Easy Chocolate Ice Cream	4	632	1.7	34	79	71	244
	1	158	0.4	8	20	18	61
Raspberry Pie	10	3844	40.7	184	519	293	1394
	1	384	4.1	18	52	29	139
Red Appleberry Pie	10	4266	33.9	181	640	302	1192
	1	427	3.4	18	64	30	119
Relish	16	562	7.3	-	142	334	1465
	1	35	0.5	-	9	21	91
Rice Custard	4	1750	19.5	80	236	682	899
	1	438	4.9	20	59	171	225
Rice Krispie Marshmallow Bars	3	718	6.0	23	124	824	172
	1	224	1.9	8	39	258	23
Rice-Stuffed Chicken	6	1370	12.0	93	123	1145	461
	1	228	2.0	16	21	191	77
Rich Almond Cookies	17	3198	37.1	197	320	2264	362
	1	190	2.2	12	19	134	22
Roast Pork with Apples and Raisins	12	3884	196.6	283	128	705	4196
	1	324	16.4	24	11	59	350
Salad Herbs	18 Tbsp	93	5.9	-	18	32	861
	1/2 Tsp	1	0.1	-	-	-	8
Salmon Patties	6	1020	104.8	55	19	336	1704
	1	170	17.5	9	3	56	284
Saucy Lemon Chicken	5	1198	86.2	47	113	667	1294
	1	240	17.2	9	23	133	259
Sauerbraten	10	2182	163.8	144	52	1130	2757
	1	218	16.4	14	5	113	276

Sausage (see Italian, Spanish and Old-Time Country Sausage)

RECIPE	Servings	Calories	Protein gm	Fat gm	Carbohy-drate, gm	Sodium mg	Potassium mg
Savory Brussels Sprouts	6	513	10.5	47	20	604	940
	1	86	1.8	8	3	101	157
Scrambled Potatoes and Eggs	3	1051	44.7	84	34	701	651
	1	350	14.9	28	11	234	217
Scalloped Potatoes	6	1348	19.2	58	191	514	1047
	1	225	3.2	10	32	86	175
Scottish Shortbread	16	3280	37.4	188	362	2249	383
	1	205	2.3	12	23	141	24
Seafood Quiche with Crab	6	2785	99.3	191	161	3028	1324
	1	464	16.6	32	27	504	221
with Shrimp	6	2802	105.8	190	161	2770	1479
	1	467	17.6	32	27	462	247
with Tuna	6	2826	112.5	190	160	2653	1509
	1	471	18.8	32	27	442	252
Seven-Minute Frosting	16	1287	7.2	-	315	140	107
	1	80	0.5	-	20	9	7
Sherried Beef Stroganoff	6	1969	107.5	123	63	852	2411
	1	328	17.9	21	11	142	402
Shish Kabobs	5	1302	89.2	86	43	473	2358
	1	260	17.8	17	9	95	472
Short-Cut Brownies	16	1592	24.2	66	259	562	600
	1	100	1.5	4	16	35	38
Shrimp and Fish Creole	5	1397	98.8	17	214	641	3177
	1	279	19.8	3	43	128	635
Shrimp Broiled with Garlic Butter	5	1244	83.5	96	12	1758	1099
	1	249	16.7	19	2	352	220
Snickerdoodles	30	4476	54.2	200	616	4305	952
	1	149	1.8	7	21	144	32
Sour Cream Pineapple Pie	10	3333	39.8	137	491	232	1042
	1	333	4.0	14	49	23	104

RECIPE	Servings	Calories	Protein gm	Fat gm	Carbohy-drate, gm	Sodium mg	Potassium mg
Sour Cream Sauce	4	439	4.0	45	6	330	107
	1	110	1.0	11	2	83	27
Southern Pecan Pie	10	4250	36.4	220	544	92	895
	1	425	3.6	22	54	9	90
South of the Border Relish	32	101	4.9	1	22	24	751
	1	3	0.2	-	1	1	23
Spaghetti Sauce	8	2235	133.5	158	70	552	4615
	1	279	16.7	20	9	69	577
Spanish Sausage	9	1116	70.0	88	5	202	827
	1	124	7.8	10	1	22	92
Spiced French Toast	6	743	33.8	23	95	1066	576
	1	124	5.6	4	16	178	96
Spiced Squash	4	304	4.2	13	46	147	759
	1	76	1.1	3	12	37	190
Spiced Tea	24	70	2.8	-	16	1	1109
	1	3	0.1	-	1	-	46
Strawberry Bavarian Cream	8	2325	28.0	97	348	148	1278
	1	290	3.5	11	44	19	160
Strawberry Bread	18	3075	29.7	145	444	673	601
	1	205	2.0	10	30	45	40
Strawberry Cream Cheese Pie	10	2654	29.4	175	243	1912	1147
	1	265	2.9	18	24	191	115
Strawberry Parfait	6	1386	9.5	45	233	5	1068
	1	231	1.6	8	39	9	178
Strawberry Pie	8	2799	18.4	84	498	10	1115
	1	350	2.3	11	62	1	139
Strawberry Sherbet	6	987	2.1	18	209	100	402
	1	165	0.4	3	35	17	67
Streusel-Topped Muffins	14	2159	34.2	81	326	1420	703
	1	154	2.4	6	23	101	50
Stuffed Cabbage Rolls	6	1789	106.3	109	93	506	3123
	1	298	17.7	18	16	84	521
Stuffed Flank Steak	8	1850	160.3	100	60	1698	3360
	1	231	20.0	13	8	212	420

RECIPE	Servings	Calories	Protein gm	Fat gm	Carbohy-drate, gm	Sodium mg	Potassium mg
Stuffed Pepper Cups	6	1859	101.4	99	136	542	3255
	1	310	16.9	17	23	90	543
Swedish Cucumbers	4	280	6.2	22	16	68	602
	1	70	1.6	6	4	17	151
Sweet and Pungent Chicken	6	2037	110.7	49	298	1005	2612
	1	340	18.5	8	50	168	435
Sweet Chocolate Cream Pie	10	2559	23.6	163	261	1643	971
	1	256	2.4	16	26	164	97
Sweet and Sour Pork	4	2123	73.9	146	130	696	1752
	1	531	18.5	37	33	174	438
Sweet 'N Spicy Dressing	1-3/4 Cups	1468	0.1	109	132	204	77
	2 Tbsp	105	-	8	9	15	6
Sweet Pickles	1 Qt.	965	8.1	1	244	59	1695
	2 Tbsp	15	0.1	-	4	1	27
Sweet Red Dressing	2 Cups	2648	2.7	218	180	955	409
	3 Tbsp	249	0.3	21	17	90	39
Tangy Coleslaw	8	693	7.2	29	101	182	1404
	1	87	0.9	4	13	23	176
Tea Cakes	16	375	31.4	187	399	2247	336
	1	211	2.0	12	25	140	21
Texas Cake	24	6095	55.9	185	1088	3114	1242
	1	253	2.3	8	45	130	52
Thumbprint Cookies	8	1709	15.9	98	194	1138	231
	1	214	2.0	12	24	142	29
Tropical Cheesecake	8	2330	23.8	146	242	1174	984
	1	291	3.0	18	30	147	123
Tuna Croquettes	8	2729	141.3	170	152	1906	2172
	1	341	17.7	21	19	238	272
Tuna Macaroni Salad	4	1807	74.7	126	94	1063	1025
	1	452	18.7	32	24	266	256

RECIPE	Servings	Calories	Protein gm	Fat gm	Carbohy-drate, gm	Sodium mg	Potassium mg
Tuna Noodle Casserole	6	2614	110.0	166	164	1749	1241
	1	436	18.3	28	27	292	207
Tuna Patties	8	736	118.4	17	19	276	1218
	1	92	14.8	2	2	35	152
Tuna Rice Casserole	6	1963	103.9	113	124	1188	1366
	1	327	17.3	19	21	198	228
Turkey Broccoli Au Gratin	6	1461	110.1	89	52	1344	1993
	1	244	18.4	15	9	224	332
Turkey Croquettes	8	2793	126.5	184	152	2120	2174
	1	349	15.8	23	19	265	272
Turkey Glory Sandwich	6	2514	111.1	169	132	2543	1236
	1	419	18.5	28	22	424	206
Turkey Noodle Casserole	6	2611	104.6	169	164	1789	1303
	1	435	17.4	28	27	298	217
Upside-Down Lemon Meringue Pie	8	2268	19.1	78	366	430	291
	1	284	2.4	10	46	54	36
Veal Coating	6	404	13.0	5	76	746	238
	1	67	2.2	1	13	124	40
Veal Goulash	6	1601	97.4	113	43	944	2100
	1	267	16.2	19	7	157	350
Veal Piccatta	3	578	58.2	38	8	362	810
	1	193	19.4	13	3	121	270
Veal with Sour Cream	6	2119	103.6	156	37	854	2162
	1	353	17.3	26	6	142	360
Vegetable Fish Bake	6	1057	93.7	52	50	120	2242
	1	176	15.6	9	8	187	374
Vienna Flavored Coffee	20	907	1.6	22	171	142	1028
	1	45	0.1	1	9	7	51
Vinaigrette Sauce	6	652	0.9	71	8	8	118
	1	121	0.1	12	1	1	20
Waldorf Salad	6	1308	3.6	124	53	1034	767
	1	218	0.6	21	9	172	128
Walnut Penuche	7	2743	13.4	65	537	346	476
	1	380	1.9	9	75	48	65

RECIPE	Servings	Calories	Protein gm	Fat gm	Carbohy-drate, gm	Sodium mg	Potassium mg
Western Gingerbread	18	3265	44.8	122	501	2958	1207
	1	181	2.5	7	28	164	67
Zippy Mayonnaise	2 Tbsp	127	0.2	13	3	82	26
Zucchini Bread	20	3124	46.0	158	400	887	1169
	1	156	2.3	8	20	44	58
Zucchini Italian Style	6	224	5.8	15	18	7	962
	1	37	1.0	3	3	1	160

INDEX

INDEX

INDEX

INDEX

INDEX

INDEX

INDEX